In My Mind

Book 2

K. Rareheart

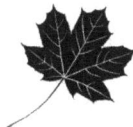

MAPLE
PUBLISHERS

In My Mind – Book 2

Author: K. Rareheart

Copyright © 2025 K. Rareheart

The right of K. Rareheart to be identified as author of this work has been asserted by the author in accordance with section 77 and 78 of the Copyright, Designs and Patents Act 1988.

ISBN 978-1-83538-534-0 (Paperback)

Published by:
Maple Publishers
Fairbourne Drive, Atterbury,
Milton Keynes,
MK10 9RG, UK
www.maplepublishers.com

Introduction

In My Mind

Book 2

This book is the follow-up to *Book 1*

(*In the Mind of a Child*)

I have titled it *In My Mind* – Book 2.

This is still a true story about the same little boy from *Book 1* (*In the Mind of a Child*), now older and facing even more traumatic times in life. I share how I overcame these challenges through my faith, my unwavering belief in God, and the positive outlook I've always held on life itself.

From a young age, I have always had a *local* mind – a practical, down-to-earth way of thinking – and this has helped me throughout my life. I've tackled many stresses and hardships along the way, although there were times when I got things wrong.

Chapter 1

The Death of My Mum

2012

My mum was 99 years old and was finding it hard to remember things, but she was always fun and loving. All her life, she had looked forward to getting a telegram from the Queen on her 100th birthday, which was in April.

In her later years, my sister looked after Mum. Every night when they went to bed, Mum would always say, "Good night and God bless," without fail. But on the last night, she was different. When they went to bed, she didn't say good night as she always did. Instead, she said, "Goodbye," as though she knew it was her time to leave this earth and be with my dad, who passed away in 1982.

My sister thought it was a bit strange at the time, but she said good night to Mum as always and went off to bed.

The next day, my sister went into Mum's room with a cup of tea. It was then that she discovered Mum had passed away. She was devastated and cried for some time before making all the necessary phone calls to let the family know the sad news.

We all made our own arrangements to travel from all over the country for the funeral. My oldest sister travelled from Scotland, and my brother, sister-in-law, nephew, nieces, my wife, and I came from

Eastbourne, Sussex. Everyone from Sussex travelled in convoy up to the Northeast of England.

We got into our cars that day with heavy hearts. I was upset, but I knew I had to pull myself together to concentrate on driving the 480 miles to our destination. Once I'd gathered myself, we set off onto the motorway.

When we arrived at a service station just outside London, we stopped for a bite to eat. None of us felt like eating much, but we needed the break. It was then that my brother and his wife realised they had left their Salvation Army uniforms on the back of the sofa at home. The look of devastation on their faces was clear. My nephew said, "I'll go back to Eastbourne to pick them up." It was a 130-mile round trip.

The rest of us carried on our journey to Darlington to my sister's house. My wife, Nikki, and I followed my brother. At one point, I said to Nikki, "What is Kevin doing?" He was driving at the national speed limit of 70 mph, but every 50 or so miles, he would slow down to 60 mph and drop behind the lorries for about 60 miles before speeding up again to overtake. Then he'd slow down once more. I said, "What's he playing at? Why doesn't he just stay in the fast lane? We'll get there much quicker at 70 mph if he does."

Nikki replied, "I don't know. Just stay behind him."

"OK, we will," I said, and that's exactly what we did for the rest of the journey.

My nephew caught up with us about 265 miles from our destination, flashing his lights and honking his horn to say, "I'm back!" We were relieved to see him. I said to Nikki, "How did he catch up so fast?"

Nikki joked, "He must have put a rocket in his exhaust pipe!" For the first time since leaving home that day, I smiled.

We arrived at our hotel to sort ourselves out for Mum's funeral the next day. In two stints, we had travelled over 850 miles practically non-stop, all to honour Mum for the life she had lived and the kindness she had shown to so many people.

The following morning, after breakfast, we went to my sister's house. About an hour later, Mum's hearse arrived. We all stood outside as it pulled up. My oldest sister went to the back of the hearse and spoke to the driver. They pulled Mum's coffin out slightly so she could straighten the Salvation Army flag draped over it. Once it was straightened, the coffin was slid back into the hearse.

Soon after, we all got into the limousines and went to the crematorium for the service. As Mum's coffin disappeared behind the curtains, we went outside, talked for a while, and made plans to meet again at the wake later that evening.

That afternoon, Kevin, Marjorie, and the kids went for fish and chips – northern style with crackling, just the way we had it when we were kids. We talked about Mum, how she had been when we were growing up, and how loving she always was.

That evening, we went to the new Salvation Army building, as the old one had been condemned years before. Nikki and I sat at the back so that if it all got too much for me, I could slip out for a cigarette without anyone noticing. During the meeting, I went out twice.

On stage, a big screen displayed the story of Mum's life and all the things she had achieved. For me, it was a huge eye-opener. I had no idea just how remarkable Mum truly was. I had been so consumed with anger and unanswered questions that I never noticed all the things Mum was doing for others. How selfish I had been, wrapped up in my own issues.

The achievements in Mum's life were incredible. She lived her life helping others, and she was an inspiration to everyone who knew her. The love and kindness she shared were endless.

After the wake, we mingled with the other guests. Some of them came up to Nikki and me and said, "Who are you?"

I replied, "I'm Kevin's brother."

"Oh," they said, "you're Brian! We haven't seen you in years."

I smiled and said, "It's been more like 40 years since I've been to Darlington." They asked if I remembered certain people from my childhood. Some I had forgotten, but others I could recall.

After the evening ended, we all went our separate ways. The next day, we had to drive back to Eastbourne.

At breakfast the following morning, Nikki said, "Can we go home via Hoveringham?"

"Where's that?" I asked.

"It's on our way back," Nikki replied. "We can see my auntie. It's only a small village; it won't take very long."

"OK," I said, and we set off.

As we drove through Darlington, I showed Nikki some of the places I used to visit as a child. Then we hit the M1 motorway. "I hope this detour won't take too long," I said.

"It won't," Nikki reassured me.

We followed the signs for Hoveringham, but before we knew it, we had driven straight through it and ended up on a completely different motorway – the M60, which took us to Manchester, the total opposite direction. We were still heading south, so we decided to keep going, hoping we'd rejoin the route to the southeast sooner rather than later.

We had been driving for 4–5 hours when I realised Nikki had fallen asleep, her head resting on a pillow against the window. Our dog was asleep in the back of the car too.

Eventually, I spotted a sign for the south, took the turning, and we headed back towards the southeast and home.

By that time, we had been travelling for nearly eight hours, and I was getting a bit tired but still felt okay to keep going for now. I knew, however, that if I got too tired, I would have to stop and rest for a while. By this time, the motorway was getting quiet, and the traffic wasn't as bad as it had been earlier. It wasn't very long before I saw a sign that said "Brighton 150 miles." I clenched my fist and muttered under my breath, "Yes!" I knew from that point it wasn't much longer until I would see the signs for Eastbourne and home.

I looked across at Nikki and the dog; they were both still asleep. I decided to pick up the pace a little, reaching 80mph, but I didn't go too mad as I didn't want to get caught speeding. I had a clean driving licence, and I wanted to keep it that way. I slowed down to 70mph, which is what I should have been doing anyway, and felt better for it. By this time, I was getting very tired after the long drive but was determined to finish the journey back home in one piece. I knew I only had less than 100 miles to go, so I carried on.

It wasn't long before I saw a sign that said "80 miles to Eastbourne and home." The road through Brighton had taken me on a slightly different route to Eastbourne, but at least we were on the way back. It wouldn't be long now. At first, I didn't recognise the route I was on, but I carried on because I knew that eventually I'd see something familiar. By now, I was really feeling the fatigue from the long drive, and I could feel my eyes starting to close. I opened the window to let some fresh air in. Nikki was still asleep but stirring slightly.

As I drove past a place we'd been to many times, called Middle Farm, I knew we were only about an hour away from home. Just at that point, Nikki woke up and said, "Where are we?"

"We're on the A27," I replied. "We're nearly home, just an hour to go."

"What time is it?" she asked.

I glanced at the clock on the dashboard and said, "It's 1am."

"What? You've been driving all this time? We left Darlington at 10am, and you're still driving!"

I thought to myself, "Well, if you hadn't wanted to go somewhere else, we could have been home over three hours ago." But I didn't say anything. I just kept driving. We'd be home in no time now.

I said to Nikki, "If we hadn't got lost, we would be home already. Never mind, not long now." I could feel the long drive taking its toll on me, and then I saw a sign that said "3 miles to Eastbourne."

"You can open your eyes now," I said to Nikki. "We're back home, just three miles to go."

"Thank God for that," Nikki replied as she woke up fully and opened the window on her side of the car.

"Oh, look!" she said in a happy but very tired voice. "I'm so glad to be back home."

We finally pulled up outside our flat, and I switched off the car engine. For a moment, it felt like the journey would never end, but now it had. I was so relieved to be home. The dog woke up as we stopped, so I took her out of the travel cage and went for a walk around the block so she could do what she needed to before bedtime.

When I got back, Nikki took the dog inside while I unloaded the car. After that, it was time for a coffee and then straight to bed. We were all shattered after that incredibly long drive.

For the next three months, we slowly started to get used to the idea that I was never going to see my mum again. It took me nearly a year to come to terms with it all, but I eventually got back to some kind of normality. As I said to myself at the time, life goes on, and time stops for no one.

But unknown to Nikki and me, things were about to get even worse. In the next six months, we would receive the worst news anyone could ever get—the news everyone dreads: the big C.

CHAPTER 2

My Fight With Cancer

2013

It was nearly eleven months since Mum had passed away, and I was just getting used to the idea that she was gone. The next time I would see her again would be in heaven, once I had passed away myself. Looking on the bright side of life, though, that was a long way off yet.

One day, I went to the loo as you do first thing in the morning, and I spotted blood in the toilet. I immediately made an appointment to see my GP. She gave me a sample bottle, and I did the sample and handed it back the same day. She sent it off and told me not to worry until the results came back. I tried not to worry, but you do. That's the nature of the human mind. I was thinking all sorts of things— was this the end of my time on earth, or what? A week later, the result came back, and it said "inconclusive, scan needed."

My GP made an appointment for me, and it arrived three days later. I thought that was quick, and Nikki, my wife, agreed. She said, "They're working fast, but it's better to be safe than sorry."

"Yes," I replied, "but this has been mega speed. In just two days, I'll find out."

Two days later, I went for my kidney scan. I was cold and expecting some massive machine with a bed to lie on. Instead, there was a young nurse standing there with a small hand device—the kind they use to scan pregnant women. At this point, I was a bit confused. The nurse told me to strip to the waist, lie on the bed on my right side, and then she started the scan.

She pressed very hard with the device. I said, "Do you have to push so hard?"

She replied, "Yes, sorry, I must get a clear picture."

So, I just put up with it until she finished. When she was done, she said, "You'll get the results soon."

I left the room, swearing under my breath, and as I walked down the corridor, the pain on my left side was intense. It lasted a week before it eased off. When I got back home that day, Nikki was waiting for me. I told her everything that had happened.

"Why didn't they do a proper CT scan?" she asked.

I replied, "How the hell should I know?"

Just five days later, I received an appointment to have a biopsy done. I wasn't quite sure what that was, so when I got there, I waited in the waiting room for about forty-five minutes before I was called in. There was a nurse and a surgeon, who explained, "First, we will numb the area, and then we'll take four thin slices of your tissue. We'll send it off to find out what it is. You won't feel a thing. It's all done by keyhole, so it will heal quicker."

Well, in they went. He was right; I didn't feel the first slice, nor did I feel the second. The third slice, I felt. And the fourth—it felt like they were pulling my kidney out! The pain was horrendous. I clenched my fists together and gritted my teeth. Then the surgeon said, "All done. We'll send this off to the lab, and we'll let you know in due course whether it's cancer or not."

I was thinking to myself, "I bet it is. What's going to happen to me next?"

Anyway, I got dressed and went back home. I was still in agony from the procedure. That day, I was in a lot of pain, and it lasted for two weeks. During that time, I was getting very worried and depressed about it all. After four weeks of waiting, I was sick with worry. I kept thinking, "Is this going to be the end of my life? Am I about to die?" I didn't know, and I was getting very frightened. I kept my thoughts to myself so that Nikki wouldn't get as worried as I was.

Then the results came back, and my worst fear came true. It was cancer.

I said to myself, "Oh my God, what else is life going to throw at me? How much can one person put up with?" This time, I had to go for an operation, something I had never experienced before.

Just one week later, I was in hospital to have the operation on the cyst they had found. When I arrived on the ward at 6 a.m., we were all told to go into a big room where all the patients were. Once we were checked in, we were shown to our beds. I was told that I was one of the first to go down for surgery.

"Great," I thought, "it'll all be over soon."

I was also thinking about my diabetic medication and taking it on time. I thought I'd be out by dinnertime. Well, dinner came and went. I waited all afternoon, and still, I was waiting. By now, I was feeling quite unwell, having already missed two doses of medication.

At 5 p.m., the evening meal was being served, and just then, they came for me. Off I went to have the operation. When we got to the operating theatre, I spotted two huge syringes. They were about six inches long, and the syringes themselves were at least seven inches. I was so glad I was going to be under anaesthetic!

Just before I went under, they removed my dentures and wrapped them in tissue. I thought, "What are they thinking? How am I supposed to eat when I wake up with tissue and denture fixative stuck to my teeth?"

They told me the operation would take about twenty minutes. It ended up lasting four and a half hours. When I woke up in recovery, I was groggy and still in pain. Back on the ward, a nurse came over and asked if I wanted something to eat. All they offered me was a dry turkey sandwich. I looked at my teeth and thought, "How the hell am I supposed to eat this?"

I couldn't get out of bed as I was still wobbly, and I was told to stay in bed until the morning. I ripped the sandwich apart and ate just the turkey by tearing it into small pieces and swallowing it. It was dry as anything, but at least I had something to eat. After that, I slowly drifted off to sleep. It wasn't a deep sleep because of the nurses chatting just outside in the hallway.

I woke early the next morning and managed to sort my dentures out, ready for breakfast. A short while later, breakfast arrived. When asked what I wanted, I said, "Cereal, toast with marmalade, and a coffee." By the time the nurse had been around the ward, I had finished eating. She looked at me in surprise and said, "You must have been hungry."

"You could say that," I replied.

About an hour later, Nikki came to see me. While she was with me, a nurse came to check my vitals and reminded me to get out of bed and do some walking.

"OK," I said, thinking, "Yes! I can have a fag."

The nurse said to Nikki, "Do you want to go to the front of the hospital to the café?"

"That's a good idea," I said.

So, I got out of bed very slowly, and we made our way down to the café by the main entrance. I had a sticky bun and a coffee. After that, we went outside, and I had about three fags. The sun felt so good on my face, warming me up nicely. Nikki and I talked for about an hour, and then we made the slow walk back to the ward.

At that point, all the pain relief I had been given was morphine, which worked well but only lasted about three hours. On the way back, I was holding my left side. Nikki looked at me and said, "Are you OK, love?"

I said that I would be fine; it's just that the painkillers were wearing off, and the pain was getting stronger. I expected they would give me something later. Nikki said, "Yes, I think so."

We stopped for a while and looked out of the window at a fight in the car park over a parking space. We stood there for a bit until the security guards came and sorted it out. Then we went back to the ward, and I sat beside the bed. A short while later, Nikki went back home. I gave her a kiss before she left and said, "Love you, as always."

I sat beside the bed for another two hours or so. By then, the pain was easing off a bit, probably because I had been sitting still for some time. The nurses came with the drugs trolley. A nurse came up to me and asked how I was doing. I replied, "Just a bit of pain." She said I could have some pain relief and gave me two Tramadol, saying, "These will ease the pain."

Then the dinner trolley came, and I had my dinner, which made me feel better. However, just after dinner, I felt a bit drowsy. About an hour later, a different nurse came with the drugs trolley and gave me two more Tramadol. By this time, I was feeling very sleepy. It was about 9 p.m., and then at 10 p.m., the drugs trolley came again, and I was given two more Tramadol. I took them, but I was so sleepy I could hardly keep my eyes open. I just laid my head on my pillow and went straight to sleep.

During the night, my wound started leaking, so I rang the bell. A nurse came in and sorted it out. I was okay after that and went straight back to sleep again.

The next morning came, and breakfast had come and gone. I was still sleepy. When visiting time arrived, Nikki came to see me. She was surprised to see me still asleep. In all the 30 years she had known me, I had never slept that late. I had always been up at around 3 or 4 a.m.

Nikki was very concerned about what was going on, so she went to the nurses' station to find out. She was told that I had been given Tramadol the night before. When Nikki heard the word "Tramadol," she let rip at the nurses and said, "Do you know my husband is diabetic? That's a very powerful painkiller!"

The nurses assured her that they would keep a close eye on me and not give me any more painkillers until I was fully awake. Nikki had no choice but to wait to see how long it would take me to come round. At that time, they had no idea just how long this would be. Nikki kept coming to see me for the next five days, and still, there was no change.

On the fifth day, I was awake but unable to speak or wake up properly. At first, my whole life flashed before my eyes, and I could feel myself getting weaker all the time. All I knew was that I had to fight to live. For the next five days, I drifted into a deep coma-like state. My body stopped moving so vigorously, and it was then that I saw a long tunnel with a small light at the end. It was moving slowly towards me and getting bigger.

At first, I thought I was seeing things. People I had known who had died appeared before me, and I could see them very clearly. It was so strange. On the fourth day, I became scared that it wasn't going to stop. I could hear the nurses and everything happening in my head at the same time.

By the fifth day, I was extremely dehydrated and had lost a lot of weight. I could hear voices on the ward, but they were just mumbling and unclear. I was then drawn back into the tunnel, and I felt as though I was floating. Something was pulling me in two directions—one way towards the light and the other into darkness. The light at the end kept getting bigger, and it was at that point that I heard a voice.

The voice said, "Brian, your time on Earth is not yet done. You have work yet to do. It's not your time." Just then, the voice repeated the same words, but the second time, it faded into the background.

At the same moment as the voice disappeared, I felt my body back on the bed. I came back into the land of the living. Nikki said, "Look, he's waking up!"

I didn't know what day it was. My mouth felt like a desert, and I was so weak, as though all my energy had been taken away. My legs felt like jelly, and I couldn't move them myself. The nurses came over and got me up very slowly. My head was spinning, and I couldn't do anything for myself. They gave me a cup of water and told me to drink it slowly. It was nice and cold. As I felt it sliding down my throat, I thought I would never feel anything going down inside me again.

Two days later, the doctors came to see me. At first, they were nice, but then one of them said, "I can't understand it. It must have been the anaesthetic."

I looked up at them, filled with anger, and said, "Bullshit! If it was the anaesthetic, I wouldn't have been in the café the day after my operation."

One of the nurses who had been on duty confirmed, "Yes, I remember him saying he was fine to go for a walk with his wife the day after his operation."

Nikki said, "You should never give a diabetic person Tramadol. It's lethal! You, as nurses, should know that."

The doctor looked at my notes at the end of the bed and said, "The lady is right. What's this? You gave him six doses in such a short space of time. No wonder he was out of it for five days! You shouldn't blame it on the anaesthetic."

With that, they all left the ward, leaving us alone.

One of the other patients said, "We all thought you were a goner, mate, for a while there."

He introduced himself. "My name's John. I'm just going to get a coffee. Do you want one?"

"Yes, I'd love one. Black with two sweeteners, please. No, make that four sugars," I replied.

John said, "I think you need the sugar, just this once."

"You're right. Make it four," I agreed.

John said, "I'll be back in a tick."

He went to the coffee machine down the corridor. When he returned, he said, "When you're well enough, I'll show you where it is."

I asked, "Do you want any money for it?"

"No, it's free. Enjoy," he said.

He went back to his bed, and I enjoyed my first coffee in five days. It was warm and went down a treat.

Nikki carried on chatting for an hour or so, and then it was time for her to go. She told me, "Do not take any more Tramadol."

I said, "Not bloody likely."

We had a kiss and a cuddle, and then Nikki went back home. "See you tomorrow. Love you," I said.

"Love you too," she replied.

After dinner, I settled down for the night, still feeling very weak. Just before bedtime, John came over to me and said he was going back to get another coffee.

"Would you like one?" he asked.

"Yes, please," I said.

When he came back, he asked, "Can I sit on your chair for a bit?"

I was in bed by that time, but I said, "Yes." He sat down in the chair beside my bed, and we had a long chat for about an hour or so. I was a bit scared to go to sleep at first, but after a while, I drifted off. And for the record, we slept in our own beds—just in case you were thinking otherwise.

The next day came, and I was feeling a bit better but still very weak. I was determined to get on top of things. One of the nurses sorted my teeth out for me, so when breakfast came, I could eat with my teeth where they belonged. I was starving after not eating for five days and felt so lightheaded I could have eaten a horse.

I heard the sound of the breakfast trolley coming, and when it arrived, I made up for lost time and had a feast. I had four Weetabix, and by the time the nurse had been around all the beds, she said to me, "You must have been hungry!"

"That's the first time I've eaten in five days," I replied.

The nurses were new to the ward and didn't know what had been going on with me, so I let it slide.

For the next two hours, I just sat in the chair beside the bed. I tried to get up, but my legs were far too weak. I looked down and noticed a little bag, like a urostomy bag, strapped to my leg. That's why I didn't feel like I needed a wee. The nurses kept coming to empty it and check if I was OK.

I asked one of them if I would be allowed outside when my wife came to see me later.

"You're too weak to walk outside yourself," she said. "We'll get you a wheelchair so you can go out for a while."

Shortly after, Nikki arrived.

"You look a bit better today," she said.

"I feel like shit," I replied, "and so weak. I tried to get up and can't move my legs. They're being very stubborn."

Nikki said, "What do you expect? They haven't been used in five days—they're weak."

"They'll get stronger as time goes on," she added reassuringly. "Soon, you'll be walking again. You'll see."

Just then, the drugs trolley came, and the nurse asked, "Do you need any painkillers?"

Both Nikki and I said, "No! Definitely not. And no Tramadol."

"I don't want painkillers from this hospital again," I added firmly. "I'll do it myself from now on with mind over matter."

The nurse shrugged and said, "Suit yourself." She looked at me as if to say, *whatever you say, clever clogs*.

Nikki had a puzzled look on her face.

"Don't look so worried," I told her. "I've done this before. I can do it again."

"How can you do that?" she asked, clearly confused.

I explained that I used to do meditation when I was younger, after the foundry accident and my motorcycle accident.

"How do you do that?" she asked.

I went on to tell her all about it—how you get your mind into a relaxed state and drift into a semi-conscious state. It's called meditation. I told her that if you go into deep meditation, it's important to come out of it slowly and to avoid being disturbed, as it could be dangerous.

"I don't think I fully understand," Nikki said, "but you seem to know what you're doing. Just be careful."

"Don't worry," I said. "I've done it many times before."

"OK," she replied. "If you're sure."

"I'm sure," I reassured her. "I'll pick a quiet time at night and do it then."

Then I said to Nikki, "I asked the nurse about going outside, and she said I could in a wheelchair."

Right on cue, the nurse brought the wheelchair to my bed, helped me into it, and said, "Go get some fresh air."

Before we left, I asked Nikki to go into my locker and get my fags. She did, and off we went.

We walked down the corridors and out into the hospital grounds. We sat down on a bench under the trees, where it was nice and cool. I had more than one fag and rested for a long while. It was so nice to be out of the ward. Apart from the traffic, I could hear birds in the trees for the first time in five days.

I still felt drained, but I was getting better—better than I had been in a long while. I started to feel a bit cold, so we headed back inside, had a coffee, and slowly walked back to the ward.

As we passed the nurses' station, I said, "I'm back!" Nikki and I went to my bed, and I sat down in the chair.

"I'm going to go now," Nikki said. "I love you. I'll see you in the morning."

"Love you," I replied. "Always will."

She kissed me and added, "No more Tramadol."

"Not bloody likely," I said. With that, Nikki went back home.

That night, when it had gone quiet and the last observations had been done, I pulled the curtains around my bed. I put the bed into an upright position, sat with my legs crossed, and began to meditate. It was painful, but I persevered until I got comfortable and let my mind relax. I kept telling myself, *there is no pain.*

I drifted into a deep, trance-like state, shutting my ears off completely, which was easy once I removed my hearing aids. I managed to stay like that for about an hour and a half. By the time the nurses' station started to get noisy again, I slowly came out of meditation. My eyes opened, and though my legs were a bit stiff, they soon came back to life.

It was about 2 a.m., so I slipped back into bed and fell asleep.

By the next day, I was feeling a lot better—still weak but stronger than before. It was day five after my long sleep.

Before breakfast, I got up, sorted out my teeth, and had a good wash. That made me feel a lot better and fresher. I was definitely getting stronger every day.

When Nikki came to see me after breakfast, I said, "Fancy going for a walk, if you're up to it?"

She agreed. I put my dressing gown on, and off we went.

"I'm just going walkabout," I told one of the nurses.

"Take it easy," she replied.

"OK. See you in a bit," I said as we walked down the corridor.

As we walked, I stopped at a window and said to Nikki, "Look down there!" Two cars were fighting over a parking space. Nikki looked and said, "What a couple of twits," as the drivers backed into each other.

"Come on," I said. "I want a fig."

"OK," Nikki replied, as we went outside to the smoking zone. We sat there for some time, enjoying the fresh air and the sound of the birds singing in the trees before anyone else got there and it became too noisy. Those were the better moments in life.

The sun came out and warmed things up, which made it even nicer. About two hours later, I said, "We'd better go back in—it's nearly time for the drugs run. This'll be good when they ask me if I want some."

"You know what? Yes," Nikki said, and we went back inside and up to the ward. Just as we reached the nurses' station, I saw the drugs trolley coming.

"See? Told you, didn't I?" I said.

"Yes," Nikki replied, and we headed back into the ward and got settled.

The nurse came over and asked, "Need anything?"

"Just my diabetic meds, thanks," I replied. She gave them to me, and I checked them carefully before taking them. By now, I was getting paranoid about taking the right tablets after what happened last time.

"What are you doing?" Nikki asked, watching me closely as I examined each pill.

"I'm just making sure I'm taking the right ones," I said. "I'm not letting them try to dope me up again."

"I don't think they'd dare do that to you again," Nikki said.

"I'm not taking a chance after last time. I'm not going through all that again for anyone—not even those dosser a**holes," I snapped.

Nikki could see where I was coming from. I was getting irate, and she said softly, "Calm down."

"OK," I said. "It's not her fault." I did calm down after a while, but it still made my blood boil. Some nurses go about things so slap-happy and think they're God's gift.

Two days later, the pain in my side was starting to ease. The meditation was helping me. I was glad I still remembered how to do it, even though I hadn't meditated for such a long time. My teacher had told me all those years ago that I was a quick learner. Mind over matter and meditation is a powerful combination if you can master it. It had helped me in the past and would continue to help me in the future. It was such a valuable skill to have.

As each day went by, I got stronger and felt so much better. I started to go walkabout on my own, and the extra cigarettes helped—they kept me calm. I enjoyed the freedom, and it was good to get away from the ward for a while. While outside, I noticed some of the other patients looking angry and frustrated about their situation. Most of them looked like they hadn't shaved or washed in months. It made me realise how lucky I was to have been brought up with a positive mental attitude.

As I headed back to the ward, I kept thinking about those patients and how they were handling their situation. Just as I was walking in, Nikki arrived. We went back to the ward together. It was nice to see her, as always.

"With a bit of luck, you should be coming back home soon," Nikki said.

"I hope so," I replied.

When we got back, Nikki asked a nurse, "Do you know how long it will be before Brian can come home?"

"When he's done a number two properly," the nurse said.

"That's stuffed it, then," I said to Nikki. "I just can't go."

"That'll come in time," Nikki reassured me. "You were out for the count for five days. It shouldn't be much longer now."

"Yes, I know. I don't need reminding. It was the worst feeling ever, fighting from the inside to get back to the land of the living when I couldn't do anything but keep trying." I paused and added, "It was so hard fighting all that time. I was so glad when I could finally hear what was going on around me for the first time in five days."

We went for another walk, hoping it would help me go to the loo properly. This went on for three days. Then, I thought that if I ate more, it might help, so for the next three days, I ate like a pig.

On the fourth day, first thing in the morning, it finally happened—I went to the loo normally. I thought, "Yes! I'll be home soon and get the hell out of this place."

I told one of the nurses, and she said, "When you've done the next one, don't flush the toilet. Just come and show us, then we'll see about sending you home."

I was so disappointed. I just wanted to go back home to my own bed.

The next day, I managed to go again. I didn't flush the chain, and I told the nurse. She came to have a look and said, "That's better—it's almost the right colour. We'll see."

Just then, Nikki arrived. I told her, and she said, "That's good news. When can you come home?"

"Not until I can prove it by doing one and showing them," I said sarcastically. "Maybe they want to measure it as well!"

Nikki looked confused for a second, then the penny dropped. She smiled, and when she stopped laughing, she said, "You could be right!"

"Come on—fancy a walk?" I asked.

"Let's go," she said.

As we walked out of the ward, I said to the nurse, "I'm going walkabout." Nikki was still smiling to herself.

Outside, she said, "All I can think of is a nurse measuring it with a ruler! I just can't get it out of my mind."

"More than likely, she'll be smelling it to make sure it's mine!" I joked.

"You might be home tomorrow," Nikki said.

"The sooner, the better," I replied.

"We'll just have to wait and see," Nikki said.

"Can we change the subject?" I asked.

"Yes," she replied. "Thinking about it puts stupid thoughts in your head. Just think—it's only a matter of days now, and you'll be home."

"Thank God," I said. I couldn't wait.

Three days later, I was discharged from the hospital with a list of dos and don'ts, what to avoid eating, and no driving for ten weeks. Boring, but needs must. Nikki went home that morning.

That afternoon, I got a taxi, left the hospital, and went home. I rang Nikki to say I was on my way.

"Great!" she said. "I'll put the kettle on."

As soon as I walked in, Nikki said the one word I'd been waiting to hear: "Coffee!"

"That's music to my ears," I replied.

"I'm on it," Nikki said. When we sat down, I said, "It's good to be back home."

"It's great you're back home," she replied, a tear in her eye. "I thought I'd lost you back then."

I gave her a hug. "Everything's OK now. I'm made of tough stuff."

After a short while, Nikki gave me another hug, but I quickly moved her hand away from my right side. She hadn't realised it was over my wound where I'd had my operation.

"Oh, I'm so sorry," she said quickly.

"It's OK. I'll live," I replied.

We decided on dinner—fish and chips, of course—and watched TV for a bit. By 12:30 am, we went to bed. The only way I could sleep was with five pillows, sitting up. I just couldn't lie down for a long time.

That night, I fell into a deep sleep for the first time in five weeks. I had a very realistic dream—I was back on the ward, fighting to get out of the coma. I heard voices from the tunnel. One voice was my mum's, and the other was God's, saying, "It's not your time yet. Your life on Earth isn't complete. You still have things to do."

When I woke up, I realised I'd had an out-of-body experience. It all made sense to me now.

The next day, when I got up, my left side was very painful, like someone was sticking knives into me. I took some of my painkillers, and they eased off after a while, allowing me to move a bit easier. After breakfast, Nikki asked, "Are you up to going into town?" I said I thought it was too soon, but maybe we could go for a short walk later.

"Okay," she said. "Let me know when you're up to it."

"Yes, I will," I replied as I held my side, waiting for the pain to ease. A couple of hours later, I said, "I'll give it a go, but we'll just go for a short walk around the houses."

I went to put my coat on, but Nikki could see I was having a bit of trouble, so she came over to me and gave me a hand.

"Thanks," I said. "That makes me feel like I'm an old man."

She smiled and said, "It's just until you feel better. You've just been through hell and back. Don't worry, you'll be better sooner than you think. Until then, take your time. We'll do things in your time, okay?"

"Yes, of course. You can use the stair lift, I'll walk down the stairs."

"Okay," I said as we went downstairs to the front door. We stepped outside and walked up the street.

"Take your time," Nikki reminded me as we walked down the path and into the fresh air. It was so good to be out and about instead of stuck on the hospital grounds. We had a country lane right next to the flat, so we took a slow walk up it.

"I know this lane so well," I said to Nikki.

"Why's that?" she asked.

"When I was just 15 years old, I used to drive tractors up and down this lane when all this land was fields. It was full of cows and sheep. Those were the good old days when the only thing you heard

31

was the wildlife, and not the hooligans you hear today, or kids kicking poor hedgehogs like footballs. That sickens me to the stomach when I see that sort of thing going on. I only wish those kids could feel what those hedgehogs can."

As we walked further up the lane, I ended up telling Nikki all about the things I did on the farm, and about the calves being born. It brought back some good memories for me and took my mind off the pain. After a while, we stopped.

As I looked into the trees, I spotted a squirrel going into its nest. I put my finger over my mouth and quietly said to Nikki, "Look up there." I pointed at the squirrel's nest. "See it?"

Nikki looked with amazement as the squirrel came out of the nest with one of its babies in its mouth. "It must be moving them," I said. "They do that when the nest has been disturbed by a predator."

We watched for a bit, then made our way back home.

"That was better than going into town," I said to Nikki.

"Yes, it was," she replied. "I've never seen anything like that before."

When we got back home, I sat back in my armchair, totally knackered. I had a coffee and flaked out. I knew this recovery was going to take a long while. As I drifted off to sleep, my mind started to think about all the things that had happened to me in my life and how, at times, God had sent me such hard tasks to deal with. I thought about how I had managed to work them out, like when my dad and daughter died on the same day, and all the times I had been knocked down but got back up again. Life had kept going, and I had gotten back on top of things—just to be knocked down once more.

Then I woke up, and Nikki asked, "Do you want a drink?"

"Yes, please," I replied. "I haven't had one since the last one."

She said, "Funny, you're feeling a bit better."

"Just a bit," I said, as she went into the kitchen to make it. I thought, *I've got a good wife in Nikki*, and for once, my feelings were right in choosing her when I did.

Just then, Nikki came in with the coffee.

"There's a change," I said. "It's usually me doing that."

"You've made me enough drinks in the past. It's time I looked after you for a change. You deserve it after what you've just been through."

We sat down and had our drinks. While drinking my coffee, I thought about all the challenges that God had sent me and how they had made me a better person. That was just the way of life, and all I could do was deal with it the best way I could and make the best of it. I didn't say anything to Nikki because she would worry too much, so I kept my thoughts to myself. After all, I had the support of a strong family around me, and all I had to do was stay strong and get through this, just like the other times. I knew I could work it out in time.

A couple of days later, I started to feel a bit more positive. I was getting stronger, but I knew I had a long way to go before I'd be out of the woods with this cancer. I would fight it all the way for as long as it took, and I'd be damned if I was going to give up and let it win—not a chance.

After another six weeks or so, I was getting on top of it. I was much stronger and getting back to normal. I must be, because I was cracking stupid jokes again, and I was going into town more, getting back to enjoying life. I still had to go for regular appointments at the hospital for check-ups every three months for a scan and results. The first four times I got the results, I was told that the tumour was getting smaller and smaller. That was very reassuring and made me feel much better.

Nikki was the best wife a man could have. I couldn't ask for a better wife. She had been full of love and support—just great.

Then, I went to the hospital, and the doctor told me that my visits would be once a year, as the tumour was now the size of a pinhead. I went back home that day and told Nikki the news. She threw her arms around me and gave me a big hug.

"I can now drive again!" I said.

"That's great news! You're nearly free of the dreaded Big C," Nikki said. "You can drive again. We must go out and celebrate."

We usually went out for a meal, and this time, Nikki said, "It's on me."

"Okay," I said, as I picked up the car keys from the dining room table. We got into the car, but then I stopped and said to Nikki, with my hand over my mouth, "How do you start the car?" I was joking, with a big smile on my face.

Nikki laughed and said, "You see that little hole just down there? You put the key in there and turn it, and the car will start."

So, I did, and said, "Wow, you're right! It does start the car." Off we went into town.

When we arrived in town, we parked near the shopping mall and went for a meal. After the meal, I said to Nikki, "I'm not over it yet, but I'm getting there. It was so weird driving after all this time."

"Yes, you are. Keep doing what you're doing," Nikki said. "I knew you would beat it. You have the willpower."

When we went back home that day, I felt like a big weight had been lifted off my shoulders, and I felt so much happier than I had in a long time. It made me feel like a winner after all. That night, I slept with the thought that my life was going to be much better from now on, with less worry than it had been in a long time. Life was going to be good to me for a change, and I was now ready for it. For once, I was ready for anything life had to throw at me.

The next morning, I felt so good that I was cracking jokes again. Nikki could see the defiance in me and said, "You're back to yourself again." "Yes," I said, "I feel so good after the news yesterday." Nikki asked, "What do you want to do today?" I replied, "What I'd like to do is go out with some sandwiches and take some photos of the wildlife." Nikki said, "We haven't done that in such a long time." So, we packed up the camera, sandwiches, and went out into the countryside to take a lot of photos.

We had a really nice, relaxing day and forgot about the big C for the day. We got some nice photos that day, and I felt even more relaxed than I had when I woke up that morning. It was so good to feel so good after all the worries of the last two years.

For the next three years, I still went to my appointments at the hospital. Five years later, I got the wonderful news that I was now free of cancer. I will never forget how I felt that day when I got the news. When I came out of the consulting room, I was all choked up inside. When I went back home and told Nikki, we were both over the moon, ecstatic with the news. I said to Nikki, "I don't believe it! I'm free. I've done it. No more cancer to worry about anymore!" I said this with my fists clenched in the air. From then on, we could move on with life and stop worrying about it.

I rang my sister-in-law to tell her, and my brother Kevin the good news. It was then that I was told that Kevin had just been diagnosed with cancer and would be starting treatment next week. That was the biggest blow of all to me. I was celebrating, and my brother was just starting chemo. I thought, *He doesn't deserve this,* and I really hoped he would pull through and fight it the way I did.

So, we wished him all the very best for the future. I told him, "I've just beaten it, and you're as strong as me. You can beat it too, just like I did." I then said that I would pray for him to have the strength to beat it as I had. I told Nikki the news, and she said, "We will be thinking of Kevin and Marjorie at this time." I said, "Why does it always seem to happen to the nice people in this life and not the nasty people? It's just not fair."

After the sad news about Kevin, it took us nearly two months to accept the news before we started to get on with our lives. Nikki and I started to plan for our future, and we could start to fulfil our plans to go out and about taking pictures of the wildlife. We made plans to go to different places to get the best pictures we could, which took us into the woods, as well as to zoos, up onto the South Downs, and many other places.

I felt free and so much happier, but at the same time, I was always thinking of Kevin and what he was going through. As for me, I had never felt so good in a long time. Life was good again, and we were both a lot happier than we had been in over the last three years.

Two months went by when I received a letter from the Cancer Association with a badge inside that said "Cancer Survivor," which I now wear with pride. There are many people who have not been as lucky as I have. They are fighting cancer all over the world, and many are losing their fight. But now, the scientists have made leaps and bounds, finding cures for many cancers. Maybe one day they will find a cure for all cancers known to mankind. There are over 250 types of cancer now, and it would be great to be able to eradicate all of them.

It has been five years since I had my operation for cancer, and I have just been for a routine check-up. I found out that when I had my operation, they removed half of one of my kidneys. So, I've been living with 1½ kidneys, which was a bit of a shock, but hey-ho, that's life.

Chapter 3

Nikki's Dialyses

2014

Nikki started to feel very ill. Her face was turning discoloured, a yellowish colour. I asked her, "Do you feel okay?" She replied, "Yes, just a bit tired. I'll be fine." I said, "Have you looked at yourself in the mirror lately?" She got up and went to the bathroom, then said, "I think you're right. I don't know why, but you're right. I have gone a strange colour. I think I'd better see a doctor." We made an appointment for the next day.

When the doctor saw Nikki, she said, "You look like you might have kidney problems." She took a blood test and sent it to the lab for testing, telling us she would let us know when the results came back.

A week later, the results were in. We were called into the doctor's office, and the news was not good. In fact, it was quite bad. The doctor told us that Nikki was in the second stage of kidney failure and would need dialysis. An appointment was made for us to visit a dialysis specialist in Bexhill, and just two days later, we went. We expected to be the only ones there, but when we arrived, we were shown into a room with twelve other people, all there for the same reason. Nikki and I sat down, and shortly after, a woman entered the room. She was dressed in an eccentric way, with bright red hair, high heels, and unusual clothing. She looked quite weird, but she introduced herself and explained that she was there to give us all the information we needed about starting dialysis.

We were moved into a larger room, warmer and more comfortable, where we sat around a big table. She handed out leaflets and explained the different methods of dialysis. First, she told us about the Pick-Line, which is inserted into your chest and attached to an internal vein, with the tube coming out of the chest. The second method was called a Fistula, where two veins are joined inside the body, and the needles are inserted on the outside. The third method was a Graft, where the graft is placed just under the skin, connecting the veins in the body, and dialysis needles are used each time. The whole thing was mind-blowing, to say the least.

After the presentation, we had a chance to ask questions. The session lasted for about an hour, and then we made our way back to the car park. Once Nikki and I were in the car, she asked, "Did you understand any of that?" I replied, "I got the gist of some of it, but the rest of it was just a load of gibberish. We'll have to read through the info and see if we can get to grips with it all. There's a lot to get through. God help us."

At the end of the meeting in Bexhill, we were given an appointment for Nikki's first operation. She had a Pick-Line put in, and dialysis started the following week. For this, we had to go to Brighton every day for two hours of dialysis, and we also had to be trained so we could do it at home.

During our first session, we were shown how to set up the dialysis machine. It was not easy to understand, and they tried to explain the different functions of the machine, but we couldn't make heads or tails of it. They also told us how much equipment we would have at home and how much space we would need to store it. It was overwhelming. After three weeks, we decided that we just couldn't get our heads around it all. It was too much. We thought it would be best to leave it to the experts and just show up for the treatments. We didn't have enough room for all the equipment anyway, and my dyslexia didn't help matters.

Nikki and I went to Brighton for her first session, which lasted four hours, three days a week. I decided it would be better for me to drop Nikki off at 6 am and return at 11 am. This way, I didn't have to spend the whole four hours waiting in the car park. I could go home and do some housework or something.

After the first week in Brighton, Nikki's Pick-Line stopped working, so she had to have a new one put in. This time, they put in a longer one, and it worked for the next two years.

We did this for about two years, then Nikki was moved to Eastbourne, which was much easier for both of us, as it was only one mile down the road from our home, not the 64-mile round trip we had been doing. The unit was temporary, made up of three artic lorries put together inside a disused unit opposite the police station. The driveway was mud, and in the winter, I had to take the car through the car wash three times a week just to keep it clean. It was a nightmare at the time, but when needs must. On the last week we were there, they put in a concrete driveway. The next week, we moved to a new unit in Polegate, just three miles away, which was much better.

After we had been in Polegate for about a year, Nikki's Pick-Line stopped working again. It was decided that Brighton would try a Fistula on Nikki, as it would be better and more long-lasting. So, Nikki and I went over to Brighton for the operation, but it didn't work. They tried three times to insert a Fistula, but each attempt failed. In the end, they put a Graft in her arm instead, but it couldn't be used straight away, so Nikki had to have another temporary Pick-Line until the Graft had matured. When Nikki came home that day, her arm was black and blue, and she was in a lot of pain. She didn't sleep well that night, and the worst part was that she had to have dialysis the next day at 7 am.

A few weeks later, they started using her Graft, and it worked fine for the next eight months. Then, it collapsed because the needles had been inserted in the same place each time, instead of in a ladder-like fashion, which caused it to fail.

So, it was back to Brighton for another operation. This time, it was decided that the best option for Nikki was to stick with the Pick-Line, but with the longest line available, as it lasted much longer—on average, 8 to 10 years. Nikki had to stay in hospital for two weeks, and I went to see her every day. During the operation, Nikki went into anaphylactic shock and had to be put on a life support machine for two days. I was told about it when I arrived at the hospital and was shocked. I asked why I hadn't been informed at the time, and all they did was apologise. I went down to intensive care and was shown where Nikki was. When I saw her, she was on the life support machine. I was in shock. They were just about to take Nikki off the machine, so I had to stand aside while they did it. It wasn't long before Nikki started breathing on her own again. Just before Nikki was taken off the machine, I was told that she had died for 10 minutes before her heart was restarted. I nearly collapsed at the news. I just couldn't believe it. I was angry that I hadn't been told at the time, but I was also relieved that Nikki was going to be okay. Or so we thought at the time. We had no idea that Nikki would end up with short-term memory loss, which would affect her for the rest of her life.

That was something I would have to contend with as time went on. I was more concerned about getting Nikki back home sometime in the near future. Just then, Nikki woke up and opened her eyes. When her eyes became focused, she grabbed my hand and asked, "Am I in heaven?" I said, "You were gone, but now you're back with me where you belong." She smiled at me and said in a croaky voice, "I love you so much."

I told her how much I loved her too. The doctor came over to me and said, "Your wife needs to rest now. Come back tomorrow. By then, she will be on a ward, so ring first to make sure." I said my goodbyes to Nikki and went back to the car park. But before I paid for the car park, I went into a corner and burst into tears. I just didn't know how much of this I could take. Life had just been one thing after another for years now.

I pulled myself back together. I had to, so I could drive home. I paid for the car park and drove out, back on the road to home. It seemed to be the longest drive back home I had ever been on. When I arrived back home, I ordered a takeaway. All I could think of was my beloved Nikki going through that horrible experience of anaphylactic shock, her heart stopping, and Nikki dying for 15 minutes before her heart was restarted and she came back to life.

I managed to eat most of the takeaway, watched a bit of TV, and then went to bed, tossing and turning all night. The next day, I went back to the hospital to see Nikki, and to my surprise, she was much better and brighter. She said she never wanted to go through that again. I said, "Neither do I. I don't ever want to see that again. Last night, I just couldn't sleep. I did get some sleep though."

The doctor came in to see how Nikki was doing and said she could come back home in two days' time. After my visit that day, Nikki said to me, "Go home and rest, then come back and pick me up the day after tomorrow, OK?"

I said, "Are you sure?" She replied, "Yes, get some rest tomorrow and I'll see you when you come back to pick me up." I said, "OK, I'll see you at 2 pm the day after tomorrow. Love you as always." Then I turned and walked away to go back home, saying, "See you soon."

The day Nikki came back home, on the way back, I worked it out and said, "Do you realise you've had 18 operations now?" Nikki said, "I've had enough now. I don't know if I can take anymore," with a tear in her eye. "Come on," I said, as I was still driving at the time, "this should be the last one for a while. You never know, you might get a transplant by the time this one stops working."

"I'm flaming well hoping so," she said as we got closer to home. She was very upset that day. When we got back home, I tried to think of something to cheer her up. I thought of a Chinese takeaway, so that's what I suggested. Nikki said, "Yes, that will be just the thing." So, I ordered it as soon as we got in, and we enjoyed it. Nikki cheered up after that. We settled down to a relaxing evening watching TV.

The next day we stayed in and relaxed. All I could do was try to make Nikki as comfortable as I could. It was hard, but worth it to see a smile on her face. The next day was dialysis again, back to the same old routine. Dialysis became a bit of a chore sometimes. It seemed to drag on and on. It was just like that's all we ever did from one week to the next, and we didn't have time for anything else.

That's when I thought, I've always wanted to take up a hobby like photography. I had just got a new camera, so I mentioned it to Nikki. She said, "That would be a good idea. It'll give us something to focus on." I said, "You can use my old camera. I'll show you how to use it. You'll get the hang of it in time." So, we started to go out on Nikki's non-dialysis days to break up the mundane routine we had gotten ourselves into. It worked. We became less focused on dialysis and more on taking pictures of wildlife, and we got quite good at it in time.

A year went by without any problems with Nikki's dialysis until Nikki's PICC line got blocked and she had to undergo another operation. We went to the hospital and I dropped her off. I was not allowed to stay, as the COVID-19 virus was now well and truly with us, and we had to stay in a lot or, when we went out, we just went to more secluded places, keeping away from other people.

Nikki had to undergo another operation the next day. We said our goodbyes. Nikki said to me, "Take care on your way back home." I just said, "Don't worry about me. I'll be OK. I'll see you tomorrow after your operation." I went back to the car and made my way back home. I rang Nikki when I got back just to let her know that I was home. She said she was OK, just a bit nervous about the operation. I said, "You'll be just fine. You've had the same one before." She said, "Yes, I know." We ended the call in the normal way and everything seemed OK. So we thought.

The next day, when I rang the hospital, they told me that something went wrong during the operation and that Nikki had been taken into intensive care. I was to get to the hospital as soon as I could. I said, "I'm on my way." My mind went into overdrive. I quickly put my shoes and coat on, went downstairs, and got into the car. By this time, my heart was racing and I was panicking, so I sat in the car for a short while to compose myself before I drove to Brighton Hospital. I took a few chances by speeding when I could get away with it. When I arrived at the car park, there was a queue. It took nearly 10 minutes to get into the car park and park.

I went straight up to the ward, knowing that intensive care was in another building. On my way to intensive care, my heart was working overtime. I was thinking, *Not again. Don't tell me another anaphylactic shock. Oh God, I hope not.* When I got there, a nurse showed me the way to the ward where Nikki was. I said, "Thanks." But what I was about to see... Nikki was in bed, with tubes in her mouth and on life support once again.

A doctor came up to me and said that Nikki had suffered a second anaphylactic shock and that she had died for 25 minutes. She had been brought back to life and would be OK now. They were just going to take the tubes out and I would have to wait outside for a while they did what they had to.

Well, you could have knocked me down with a feather. As they took the tubes out, Nikki coughed as if she was choking. I had tears in my eyes and down my face. I was thinking that I had lost her, but just then Nikki opened her eyes, still coughing a bit. At first, she was a bit disoriented.

Soon after that, the doctor said to me, "It's okay now, you can come in." So, I did. When Nikki saw me, she burst into tears, which set me off. We gave each other a big hug, and when we had calmed down and pulled ourselves together, we realised just how lucky we were to still be alive. We looked around at all the other people there, so close to death's door, and we thought about how lucky we had been. The doctor said that Nikki should be able to go home in the next day or two. They took Nikki out of the Acute Care Unit (ACU) the next day and put her back on a ward, where she got some rest. Three days later, we would be going home soon, but Nikki had to stay in hospital for another week before she was allowed back home.

Just over a week later, I went back to the hospital to bring Nikki home. As we left the ward and walked down the corridors to the exit, we stopped by the vending machines and got some snacks for the journey back. Nikki told me all about what had happened, and I was shocked when she told me. We got back to the car, drove out of the car park, and took a slow drive home. The traffic wasn't too bad, and we got back home in about 1½ hours, which wasn't too bad for that journey. We went indoors, and I got Nikki settled in. I cooked her dinner, but she wasn't up to eating much. She apologised for hardly eating, and I said, "It doesn't matter, you've just been to hell and back. It's to be expected. Maybe you'll feel a bit better tomorrow." I made her a cup of tea. Nikki said, "Thank you. You're so good to me, I love you." I said, "I love you too," and then we watched some TV until bedtime. I got a load of pillows to make

Nikki comfortable, and we tried to go to sleep, but we ended up having a bad night. I expected that. The next morning, Nikki had dialysis again, so it was an early start. After dialysis, when I went to pick her up, we just went back home and stayed in for the rest of the day.

Three weeks later, I started to notice that Nikki was forgetting things. Just small things to start with, like when she was talking, she would forget what she was saying. She got confused and would say, "Remind me of something," and when I reminded her later, she'd say, "What are you on about?" with a blank expression on her face. Sometimes she would forget what she had for dinner the night before, or whether she had taken her medication. So, I had to keep an eye on her. Life became quite hard for both of us. For Nikki, it was extremely frustrating. This was the way life was, and how it was going to be from now on.

As the weeks and months went by, we found out that this was all part of having an anaphylactic shock, and we would just have to learn to live with it. Although it was frustrating at times, we came to terms with it, and it became just part of our lives. Nikki started to make a joke of it all.

About six months later, we started to go out taking pictures of the wildlife all around us. It was very relaxing and gave us peace of mind. It was so good to have something else to focus on, apart from dialysis all the time. It brought a lot of peace into our lives. Nikki was feeling better in herself, and the peace and quiet did us both the world of good. She wasn't tired every time she came off dialysis, like she used to be. No more going back to bed because she was tired. She now had a new lease of life and more energy. It was so good to see it in her. For the next year, I kept Nikki in a routine, and she started to remember the things she had to do, and when. Soon, she was doing things for herself, which was great for me to see, and she was much more confident in herself.

Nearly four years went by until her line stopped working, and she had to have it changed again. As I took her back into hospital for her PICC line to be renewed, I could see she was getting very worried about it—the thought of being put under again, after what happened the last two times. I told her that they wouldn't make that mistake again. Nikki said, "I bloody hope not, because I'll sue them if they do." As we got closer to the hospital, Nikki seemed to calm down and was more relaxed. I took her to the ward and settled her in. Then I was told to go and settle down; she was going to have her operation the next day.

I gave Nikki a quick kiss and cuddle, saying, "You'll be just fine. I'll ring you in the morning after your op, okay?" She nodded, and as I turned to go back to the car park, I prayed to God that she would be okay. I said, "Of course, I will," and then I took a moment and prayed again for Nikki's safety. I started the car, pulled out of the car park, and made my way home. It was 5 pm when I left the hospital, and the traffic was horrendous, so it took me a lot longer to get back home.

I stopped at the local fish and chip shop for dinner and took it back home. I was a bit late that day taking my medication, but I got away with it. I didn't feel dizzy, so that was okay. I had my fish and chips, enjoyed it, watched some TV, and went off to bed quite late.

The next day, Nikki was due to have her operation, so I rang in the afternoon to see how she was doing. When I rang, Nikki had had her operation and was doing just fine. She could come back home the next day, all being well. They just had to check her new line, and after that, she could come home. We looked at each other and smiled. I said, "See? I told you that you'd be just fine." Nikki replied, "You can understand why I felt that way." I said, "Yes, of course," as I put my arm around her. "Just think, this time tomorrow you'll be back home where you belong." Nikki said, "I can't wait."

The next day, I drove back to the hospital to pick Nikki up. When I got there, Nikki was up, dressed, and ready to go. She was a bit sore from the operation but okay. I picked up her case, and we went back to the car and headed home. It took Nikki some time to get over the operation, but after a while, when Nikki was better, we got back to some kind of normality. We got back to photography, made new friends in the world of photos, and I had managed to save up for a new camera. I gave Nikki my old one, which was still in very good condition. We started to be happy once more. For the next three years, things were very good. We started to go to zoos to get pictures of wild animals. We went as far as Hewlets in Kent, which was a 2½-hour drive by car. It was a very early start, and we were very

51

tired by the time we got back home, but it was such an enjoyable day. It made us feel like we had got our lives back.

At the time, we had quite a lot of debt, just like everyone else in this life. But I had worked out how to get out of debt once and for all, even though it would take a long time. But I was determined to do it by the time I retired. And one year before I retired, we did it. It felt so good, and now we could do some serious saving, which helped us feel ready for retirement. The pressure was lifted off our minds.

What annoyed us was the increase in phone calls saying they could help with all our debts. When we said we had no debt, they didn't believe us. So, in the end, we just put the phone down on them. I even pulled over once to take one of these stupid calls, but I made a new policy: If my phone rang when I was driving, I would just ignore it. If it was important, they would ring back.

Chapter 4

My Diabetes

2015

With all the stress I've had in my life, I've been so busy looking after Nikki over the years that I didn't realise I had been neglecting myself. I was now four stone overweight. My weight had always been around 10-10½ stone since I was about 16 years old, but now I was feeling very tired all the time. I struggled to get up in the mornings, and all my get-up-and-go had all but gone. I just couldn't understand why I was feeling this way. Life had become too much for me to bear.

Nikki had noticed and, on more than one occasion, said that I looked very ill and that I should make an appointment with the doctor. So, I did. I went to see my GP, and she took a blood sample and sent it off to the lab. She said we would know the results in a week's time and that I should make an appointment to see her then. I made an appointment for a week later.

Over the next few days, I thought long and hard about why I had gained so much weight. Then, I realised that the reason could be all the pasties, pork pies, cakes, fish and chips, and all sorts of things like that, with not enough exercise. I just couldn't put my finger on it.

A week later, I went to see my GP, and she told me that I was type 2 diabetic. That was a bit of a shock to me, to say the least. Just the thought of it brought back memories of my stepdad, who was diabetic towards the end of his life. I thought this was the end for me, but my mind was running away with me. The doctor reassured me that it wasn't a death sentence; it could be managed with diet and exercise. At first, I was very confused, but the doctor reassured me that it was controllable by diet and avoiding sweet things. She gave me a list of things to avoid and put me on a lot of new medication. She said I would see her again in a month's time.

On the short walk home, I thought hard and made up my mind that I was going to do this religiously. I had to, and I was determined to get on top of this. When I got home and told Nikki, she looked at me and said, "Bloody hell, don't worry. We can do this together. Good job we're shopping tomorrow!"

The very next day, when we went shopping, it took us three hours, where it normally took about an hour at most. We looked at every label, saying, "Can't have that," or "I can have this." We were getting funny looks from other people shopping, but I said to Nikki, "Don't bother about them. We've got our reasons."

By the time we finished, we were both tired, so we went straight home. While we were putting the shopping away, we threw out all the stuff I couldn't have anymore. We were both amazed at how much I couldn't have. I said to Nikki, "We'll get on top of this if it's the last thing I do."

Nikki said, "It will get easier as we go along. We'll get to know all the things you can have and what you can't have. Good job I can get the hang of things quickly, isn't it?"

I said, "We must start how we mean to go on."

"Yes," she said, as we filled the kitchen bin to the top. We had a cup of coffee after that, and it was my first coffee with no sugar—just two sweeteners. It was gross to me after having three sugars in every cup, but I suppose I'd get used to it in time. I was surprised at how quickly I got used to it. Within a week, I had got used to it. Before I knew it, I wasn't using sweeteners in my coffee when I was out and about either. It was very hard for me to come to terms with, but I persevered with it for a month until I went to see the doctor again. By this time, I was feeling so much better than I had a month ago.

I went to see my doctor, and she told me to get on the scales. When I did, I was very surprised: I had lost a massive three stone in just four weeks! Even the doctor couldn't believe it. She said, "How did you do it so quickly?"

I said, "I just cut out all the junk like you told me to four weeks ago and stuck to it."

"Well done," she said. "I can now refer you to the diabetic nurses for your future treatment." Then I got up and walked out the door and went back home.

I told Nikki the news, and she was a bit jealous because she had been trying to lose weight for some time so she could have a kidney transplant. She has a living kidney donor now, who is a perfect match for her, but Nikki has to lose another two or three stone first. Still, she was very pleased for me.

It was amazing how much better I felt. I had so much more energy, and all my get-up-and-go had come back. It was a great feeling to be back where I was 6 or 7 years ago. It was then that I realised just how much I had been slapdash with the things I had been eating over the years and how, if I had kept going the same way, I would have ended up killing myself. Still, I didn't, so that's a good thing—I'm still here to tell the tale.

Meanwhile, Kevin's cancer was getting better, and he was not feeling so tired. He had always been strong-minded and strong-willed, and he was getting back to his normal joking self. He was looking forward to better times and was planning a holiday for the next year. As for me, I was getting used to my new way of life as a diabetic. It was hard at first to come to terms with it all, but after six months, when I went into shops, I had learned what I could and couldn't have. It was getting easier as time went on.

I reached the stage when we went shopping, I would walk past the stuff in the shop, and instead of picking it up and putting it in the trolley, I would say to myself, "No, put it back." The more I did that, the better I got at it, until I was doing it naturally. It's something you get used to after a while.

Nikki said, "It's great how you've taken diabetes all in your stride."

I said, "It could be that I have a good memory and pick things up more easily than you do, but I've had a lifetime of practice with my dyslexia. I've had to learn from an early age how to recognise pictures and match them to what the words mean."

Nikki said, "So that's why you have such a logical mind?"

"Yes," I said. "It took me a long time to get used to it, but by the time I was about 12 years old, I had got it down to a T. I suppose it's just something I've gotten used to over the years. It's always been a way for me to cover up the fact that I'm dyslexic."

I got news from Marjorie that Kevin had just been diagnosed with two more types of cancer, so he was now dealing with three types of cancer. I said to Marjorie, "No one deserves that." At the end of the phone call, I said, "All the best, Kevin is a fighter. I just hope he has the strength to beat it," and then I added, "We will pray for him." I put the phone down in shock. I just couldn't believe it. I was thinking, why Kevin? What had he ever done to deserve this?

As I sat down, Nikki looked at me and said, "What's wrong? You look like you've seen a ghost or something." I was all choked up, finding it hard to say a thing at first. I pulled myself together and said, "It's Kevin. He's just been diagnosed with two more types of cancer, on top of the one he's been fighting for the last two years."

Nikki said, "Oh my God, as if he hasn't had enough going on in his life, and now this as well?" I replied, "I can't believe it. He doesn't deserve it. He's always been a good, hard-working person, kind-hearted to everyone he's ever come in contact with in his life, and now this. I just hope and pray he has the strength to get through it."

"So do I," said Nikki, as she got up to make another drink.

I didn't sleep very well that night, nor for the next three weeks. The worry weighed heavily on me, but I eventually came to terms with it all. I was still Nikki's full-time carer, always doing the best I could for her. Even though at times I forgot about myself and my health, I managed to get back on track. My health had gone downhill for a while, but I always got myself back to full health again. Nikki always came first.

Chapter 5

The Car Accident That Changed Our Lives

2019

I am classed as a disabled driver because I drive with a steering ball, as I cannot hold the steering wheel with both hands. This is due to a motorbike accident in 1973, which left me with a weak left arm. Despite this, it hasn't stopped me from doing most things in life. It's just something I've got used to over the years. Although I don't consider myself disabled, I always say there are a lot worse off than me. I've had a couple of car crashes since then, and it's not the first time I've had a whiplash injury, which I've gotten over before. So, I know what it feels like.

But in early November 2019, little did we know how our lives would change by the end of that month. We were very happy with life as we carried on with our wildlife and pond watch, keeping an eye on the wildlife and educating people on the best way to care for them and what to feed them. We met a lot of nice people and some not-so-nice ones. Some people had a bad attitude towards life and got very angry. One young man even threatened to throw me in the pond. I just let it go, and he walked away. I think he was on drugs or something—he was as high as a kite.

In November that year, I picked Nikki up from her dialysis one day, and she was feeling very good. I suggested we go out for a meal at the harbour where all the posh restaurants are. She agreed, saying, "Why not? We haven't been there for some time." We went back home so Nikki could get changed, then went to the harbour for lunch. After lunch, we planned to go to the park. However, we didn't make it there. On our way to the park, we had a car crash that would change our lives forever.

The crash in 2019 involved a side impact, which made our car spin sideways. My immediate reaction was to grab the steering wheel with both hands and pull it hard to the left to correct the impact and prevent the car from rolling over. I managed to keep the car going straight. After the crash, I first checked Nikki's pick-line. Thank goodness, it wasn't damaged. I took all the details of the other driver, then took Nikki to A&E to get checked out, while I went to the garage to get the car seen to. They told me to contact the insurance company, but before that, I went back to the hospital to see how Nikki was doing. When I arrived, Nikki was being attended to, so I waited in the waiting room for her to come out.

I didn't have long to wait. She came out and told me that her dialysis line was okay and not damaged. I said, "That's a blessing," but it had been badly bruised, and it would take a long time to determine how it would affect her. Apart from that, she was shaken and in shock, but she was okay.

All I could think about was Nikki and how she was doing, with not a thought for myself. I just assumed all I had was another whiplash injury, and that was all that was wrong with me. I didn't get checked out by the hospital because I thought I only had a whiplash injury. But about two weeks later, I was in quite a lot of pain with my neck. The pain was the same as I had experienced before with whiplash, but this time it was a lot more severe than before. Still, I kept going, continuing my role as full-time carer for Nikki, as I had done for the last 20 years. Even though the pain was getting worse, I had to have seven pillows to prop me up in bed so I could get some sleep.

It wasn't until February 2020 that I went to see my GP. By that time, I was in so much pain I was finding it very hard to get out of bed and had to sleep sitting up. My GP sent me to the hospital for an x-ray, and I'll never forget the moment when the two young women doing the x-ray came out of the booth. They said, "Jeez, look at that!" They told me, "Don't move. Whatever you do, don't move. We need to see the doctor about this." I stood very still, not moving a muscle until they returned.

What they had seen was a slipped disc and a fractured vertebra that had healed over the time since the accident. By the time I had the x-ray, three months had passed, and the pain had calmed down a lot. I was able to move around much easier than I had in the previous three months. I had been in so much pain during that time that at times I couldn't move at all. Later, I found out that I had trapped nerves in my neck and damaged my muscles in my shoulder. No wonder I had been in so much pain!

When I told Nikki about it, she said, "No wonder you could hardly move all that time. I shouldn't have put so much on you. I'm so sorry," with a tear in her eye. I said, "It's okay. If I had realised, I would have gone to see the doctor sooner and not put up with all that unbearable pain." I added, "Now I'll just have to live with it for the rest of my life." What a numpty I'd been, stupid and stubborn! From time to time, it flares up and causes me a lot of pain, but I've learned to live with it. Thank goodness for mind over matter.

The other driver was banned from driving, and his car was written off. He had been showing off with his girlfriend in the car. They had an argument on the roadside, and she said she would never drive with him again. "Look what your stupidity has done to others!" she said. She got that right—she broke up with him right there on the roadside that day.

Our car, on the other hand, was repaired after a long time off the road. It took about four months in all, but at least we were still on the road with a courtesy car, and I could still take Nikki to all her appointments. For the next two years, we got on with life, slowly getting back to some kind of normality, even though I now had back, neck, and shoulder pain from time to time. On those days, I was unable to drive, so we stayed in some of the time, just going out for short walks. Thankfully, this wasn't too often, and as time went on, I got back to full-time driving. I was put on more medication for my shoulder, and I must take painkillers for the trapped nerves in my neck. It's more tablets for life, but after a year, I came off the painkillers and returned to living a normal life again.

However, I still have good days and bad days, and on top of that, one of my legs gets painful when I walk too far, which is giving me a bit of a problem as well. Like I need that, right? What more will I have to put up with in my life? Some of it is wear and tear as I'm getting older, with all the heavy lifting I've done in my life. All I can do is live with it. I've just about got used to it now. My life has changed from what it was, but I've managed to learn to do things differently now. I've had to slow down and not rush around so much.

By now, my neck and shoulder were causing me so many problems. I was finding it hard to do the things I used to, like using the lawnmower. The vibrations from the lawnmower were vibrating in my arms and exacerbating the pain in my neck and shoulder. So, I had to get a neighbour to help me out with the lawn, but it cost me £10 a time. It was okay until I could do it myself, which took nearly three more months. I was also finding it very hard to do the shopping, so the way around that was to not fill the bags up too much. That was the solution to that problem. All in all, we found all sorts of ways to make my life easier, and gradually, things got easier.

It took a very long time before things got back to some kind of normality. I thought things couldn't get any worse than they had been over the last 10 years or so.

Chapter 6

The Cancer That Took My Brother Kevin

2020

It was now 2020. Just when I thought that nothing else could go wrong in my life, it had. We already knew that Kevin had cancer, but by this time, he had been diagnosed with three different types of cancer, much more aggressive than the first two. We were all devastated by the news, but Kevin seemed to take it in his stride at first. He was told that he couldn't have both therapies at the same time, as it would be too much for him to bear. So, he started on the chemotherapy, just like before, and he would have the radiotherapy later, after the chemotherapy had finished.

When the chemotherapy ended, he had become quite weak, and he said to us that he could not go on with it all. I said to him, "We Loftus's are made of strong stuff, and nothing that life can throw at us is beyond solving. That's the way it's always been for us, hasn't it?" Kevin said, "Yes, you're right," with tears running down his cheeks. I went on to say to him, "Come on, I've beaten cancer, haven't I? So will you." Kevin then said he was tired. I said, "Okay, I'll leave you to sleep. I'll see you soon." With that, I left and went to walk out the door. I said to his wife, "I will pray for him." His wife thanked me as I walked down the garden path and out the gate.

When I got home that day, I said to Nikki that Kevin did not look very good at all, and I just didn't know if he would be able to pull through. Nikki gave me a hug, and then we talked about it for a long time. It was getting late, and Nikki had dialysis the next day. She was a bit tired, so she went to bed. I said I was going to stay up for a bit. We said goodnight, and she went off to bed.

I stayed up for a long time, just sitting in my armchair with a coffee and the TV off, in the peace and quiet with no traffic outside. I prayed like I had never prayed before. I said to God, "Why does all this have to happen to Kevin? He is a very good person and has been all his life. He has always been there for others less fortunate than himself and has done a lot of good things for countless other people. He doesn't deserve this." I was getting very tired myself, so I went off to bed. That night, I tossed and turned in bed all night. I just couldn't sleep at all, so I ended up getting up. It was about 2 am, but that wasn't unusual for me. I made a coffee and knew that Nikki would be up at 4 am when the alarm went off. When Nikki got up, I didn't say anything about me not being able to sleep. I just acted as normal. Nikki had enough on her plate without me making it worse for her.

The rest of our morning went as normal for a dialysis day. At 4 am, Nikki got up and came into the front room, still half asleep. At 5 am, we had breakfast and got ready to go on the dialysis run. Then I would take Nikki to the place where she had her dialysis, drop her off, and then go back home. Four hours later, I would pick Nikki up from dialysis. During those four hours, I would stay at home and catch up with the housework, as I am now retired and time is my own. But now, the only thing on my mind was Kevin and whether he would be strong enough to survive the cancer the same way I did. I really hoped he would. I kept praying hard, as he was my brother, and we had been inseparable all our lives.

When we got back home after picking Nikki up from dialysis that day, we went out into town, did a bit of shopping, and had something to eat while we were out. We had a nice time because Nikki felt so good for a change. But when we got home that day, we had a phone call from Marjorie, Kevin's wife, telling us that Kevin was back in hospital and had taken a turn for the worse.

Kevin stayed in hospital for some time, and then he was given a choice: to go into a hospice or go back home. He wanted to go home. We were told that Kevin had just two months to live. We were all extremely shocked by the news, and all we could do was make Kevin as comfortable as we could. We were all saddened, and with heavy hearts, although we kind of knew this was coming, until now we didn't know just how much more time we had with Kevin. But now we did. The Macmillan nurses were great with Kevin. They were there 24/7, which enabled us to get on with our lives as best as we could, considering what was going on with Kevin. None of us were looking forward to the time when Kevin's life would come to an end. We were all just about to find out that the two months we were told was wrong.

Just two weeks later, Kevin sadly passed away. We were all shocked when he did. We all thought we would have longer than that with him, but it was not meant to be. I didn't see him in the last two weeks of his life. I just couldn't see him so weak towards the end. Maybe I'm gutless, I don't know, but I have regretted it ever since.

Unfortunately, at the time of Kevin's passing, the COVID-19 pandemic was upon us, and no one could have a wake after someone had died. So, we had to postpone it for a long time. I said to Marjorie that I would donate £500 towards it when we could have it. Marjorie said, "That's very kind of you, Brian. Are you sure?" I said to her, "It's my pleasure. It's the least I can do. I will put the money by for you in a safe place until you want it. Just let me know." Marjorie said, "Thank you very much," and we just left it at that.

We all got on with our lives until the funeral, just as Kevin had told us. Kevin used to work for the Post Office, and on the day of the funeral, all the Post Office van depots closed for an hour while they did a convoy of respect into the cemetery, tooting their horns as a mark of respect for Kevin. That took about 15 minutes.

Nikki and I arrived just after and parked in the cemetery car park. As we got out of the car, there were people waiting for Kevin's coffin to arrive. The Salvation Army flag bearer was also there. I knew a lot of the people from the Army, as I was brought up in it as a child.

When Kevin's coffin arrived, the flag bearer went in front of the hearse and walked slowly down to the doors of the chapel where we had the service. We all went in and sat down, and a lot of people had a lot of very good things to say about Kevin, some of which even I didn't know about. I was not that surprised, knowing Kevin as I did. After the service, we all gathered outside to say our last goodbyes. While I was outside, I couldn't hold the tears back any longer, and they started to roll down my face. My niece was standing next to me, handed me a tissue to wipe my eyes, and put her arm around me to comfort me. She said, "At least he is with Aunt Elsie now. That's our mum, who died in 2012." "Yes," I said, as I got myself back together. I thanked her and had a chat for a short while. Then she had to go, as she was going back to Darlington that night. She was a schoolteacher and had to be back to work on Monday.

Nikki and I made our way back to the car and drove out of the cemetery. Instead of going straight home, we went for a drive, had a coffee, and then went back home. I was relieved in a way that Kevin was no longer in the pain he had been in, but at the same time, I was deeply saddened that I would never see him again. It was very hard for me.

Kevin and I had always been so close; he had been such an important part of my life. We had been through so much together, and we made a pact that we would always be there for each other, no matter what. We kept to it all our lives.

Over the next few weeks, which turned into months, and now, 18 months later, I miss him so very much, and I always will. But like Kevin said after he died, "When I'm gone, remember life goes on, and you must live your life to the full." He was right. The world and time will always go on. We might come and go, but time goes on, and it always will. Those were the final wise words he said.

May Kevin always rest in peace.

Chapter 7

My Stroke

September 2021

My early morning routine has always been the same. I always got up before Nikki did. I liked it that way. I would make a coffee and sit in my armchair to wake up in the morning with no radio on, just total peace and quiet, with only the sound of the birds outside singing in the trees.

But this one morning was different. I had just made my first coffee and sat down in my armchair, just the same as every day, but something didn't feel right. It's very hard to explain, but I felt a bit unsteady on my feet. When I picked up my coffee, my left hand had gone weak, so I picked it up with my right hand instead. I went and sat down with my coffee, and when I went to have a drink, my mouth wouldn't close properly. The same thing happened when I went to have my first fag of the day; I just couldn't shut my mouth. I said to myself, "What the hell is going on?" But when I spoke, it came out all wrong, and my speech was slurred. By this point, I went into the bathroom and looked in the bathroom mirror. My face had dropped on one side.

I thought about the advert I had seen on TV the night before and then thought, "Oh no, I'm having a stroke." I tried to wake Nikki, but she was dead to the world. So, I let the cats into the bedroom, and they woke Nikki up. When she came into the front room, she asked, "What's wrong?" I said, as best as I could, "I think I'm having a stroke." She looked at me with a worried expression and said, "Your face has gone down on one side. We'd better ring 999." So, we did. It took just five minutes before the ambulance arrived. They checked me over and confirmed I was having a stroke. I was taken to the hospital with the sirens blaring and the blue lights flashing. It was very frightening for me; I had no idea what was going to happen next.

Day 1

When we arrived at the A&E department, I was rushed into a bay where they checked me over and did a lot of tests. In a short space of time, they confirmed it was a mild stroke. We were wise to ring 999, as it could have been a lot worse. I was assessed and put on a ward, where I was settled in. The nurses checked on me, and one of them took note of all the medication I was on. I told her that I had Type 2 diabetes, and it was important that I had my meds on time. I've always been very specific about that since I was diagnosed, but I don't think she could understand what I was saying because I couldn't talk very well. It was just a load of mumbling. Even I couldn't understand myself. I was so frustrated, and I felt so vulnerable and confused at the time. I didn't know what was going to happen to me next or how it was going to affect me in the long term.

But my routine with my meds was about to be turned upside down. I was admitted at about 10 am, and at dinner time, the nurse came to give me my meds, but she got it wrong. I had to tell her which ones I needed. I was feeling a bit disorientated to say the least—my head was all dazed, and my coordination was out of sync. I was also having trouble controlling my movements. Walking and moving my arm felt very heavy, and I had become so slow in doing things. I was in a ward with three other men. They seemed to be okay, quite chatty with each other, but I found it very hard to speak to them or anyone else. I couldn't put a sentence together that made sense. My speech had become so bad, and it was very hard for me to talk at all. It was so strange and frustrating, and it made me feel so embarrassed. Normally, I couldn't shut up if I wanted to, but now that was all gone. I had gone completely quiet, just like I was back in my school days as a child. I just kept very quiet so I didn't get in the way. But I soon realised that we were all in the same boat. I did get used to the idea after two or three hours, and then I settled into the fact that I wasn't alone. The four of us started chatting after a short time, even though it took us quite a long time to get the words out. We all waited until we had finished trying to say something, so we could understand what we were saying to each other. Then, it wasn't so bad. The four of us started finishing off what the others were saying, and it was quite funny at times.

Day 2

The next day, when we all woke up, I had a wash and shave. One of the nurses came to give us a drink of tea or coffee. I had a coffee, and we all started chatting about ourselves. One of the men was a war veteran and had a synthetic leg, and the other had had a very hard life indeed. So, you could say we were all from different walks of life. We became good friends while we were there and got on well with each other. It was quite strange how we all just got on with each other, considering we were all there for the same reason. Soon after we had drunk our coffee, breakfast arrived, and we could have as much as we wanted. The other two had a feast, while I just had two Weetabix because I was having trouble with my mouth closing properly. I was dribbling like a baby when I was eating, and it made me feel like a baby all over again. It was so embarrassing to me, but the others didn't take any notice of it. They had all been through it themselves when they first arrived in the hospital. One of the men said, "Don't look so worried. We've all been there. It will get better, you'll see. It won't last long." I said, "I hope not." They reassured me, saying, "You'll be okay." One of them winked at me, as if to say, "You're with friends here, and we won't take the mick out of you, so don't look so worried. You'll be just fine, just give it time."

Later that day, the physiotherapist came to see me. After a long chat, it was decided that I would be better off with a walking stick to help with my balance. She said she would be back with one. A little while later, she returned with the walking stick. She adjusted it to the right height for me and then watched me use it to see if it was better for me. After that, she left me to it. I went to the toilet and felt a bit safer. I thought, "Nikki's not coming for another hour or so, so I'll see if I can go to the front of the hospital on my own and have a fag." I went to the nurse's station and asked if it was okay. They said, "Don't go too far." I said okay and walked away from the station, thinking to myself that I would take it very slowly. But I only got as far as halfway down the corridor before I turned back to the ward. I sat down on a chair beside the bed for a while until Nikki arrived. I had been sitting there for about an hour when Nikki came to see me. She was surprised to see that I was using a walking stick. I told her it was because I wasn't very steady on my feet and my balance was all over the place. I told her I wanted to go outside for a bit. She said, "I can guess why—you just want a fag." I said, "I've been in here for two days now, what do you expect?" By this time, I was getting very frustrated and angry. Nikki said she would ask one of the nurses, so she went to the nurse's station just outside the ward. They said yes, as long as Nikki went with me.

Nikki came back into the ward and said, "Yes, you can, but you'll have to take it easy." I replied, "Okay, let's go." As we left the ward, I turned to the nurse and said, "See you later." With that, we began a very slow walk out of the hospital. It took me about half an hour to get to the front of the hospital, but I did it. I stepped outside, where there were some benches, and had a well-deserved fag or three while enjoying the fresh air.

I stayed outside for a while, relishing the fresh air and the chance to get away from the ward for a bit. It was so nice. While I was sitting outside, I saw some of the other patients coming out for the same reason. Some of them looked in worse states than I was, but somehow, they looked a little better on the way back in. I could relate to that—a bit of fresh air and a change of scenery made me feel a bit more refreshed.

After some time, I thought it was time to head back to the ward. I got up and made my way back, taking a slow walk. When I got back, one of the nurses asked, "Where have you been?" I said, with great difficulty, "I just went for a walkabout. It took me a bit longer than I thought." She replied, "It's okay, it's good for you. It will help with your recovery. Just let us know next time." Nikki added, "I said I did before I went." A nurse in the background confirmed, "He did." The other nurse said, "That's okay." With a smile on my face, I said, "I'm going back to bed for a while."

I thought to myself, *I can have a fag more often now,* which made me feel a lot better. I had been craving a fag for the last two days. Nikki stayed with me for about 40 minutes. She sat in the chair beside my bed, then said, "You look a bit tired." I replied, "Yes, I am." She said, "I'll leave you for now. Love you." "Love you too," I said. As Nikki got up, she gave me a kiss and said, "I'll see you in the morning," before heading home. I went off to sleep for a while.

When I woke up, I went to the toilet, and a nurse asked me if everything was okay. I said that I was fine and that I might go for a little walk down the corridor to stretch my legs. She said, "That's okay, it's good to see you trying to help yourself." So, I went to my locker, got my fags out, put them in my dressing gown pocket, and went for a walk outside for a fag. It felt great.

While I was outside, I thought long and hard about how things would be from now on. I decided that, from now on, I was going to slow down and stop rushing around the way I used to. I went back into the ward for the night and had a good night's sleep for a change.

Day 3

The next day, when I woke up, I felt different. I felt like my life had changed. I was going to be different from now on, and all the past was now behind me. From now on, I had to live like an old man. The rest of my life was going to be this way—really slow. It would be like living my life in slow motion. In a sense, I was looking forward to a life with a much slower pace because I had been living life in the fast lane and on the edge for years. It had been a full-time career for my wife, Nikki, since she had to go on dialysis for the last seven years. Now, it had become too much at times. But, as you do with a loved one, you just plod on with life, no matter what comes your way. That's life.

Anyway, Nikki came to see me just after breakfast and said, "Fancy going for a walk outside?" I said, "I thought you'd never ask." So, we took a slow walk to the front of the hospital and sat on one of the benches for a while, talking about how things would be from now on.

I said, "I've been told I need to learn how to slow down. There will be no more rushing around like I used to, so that's just what I intend to do from now on." Nikki said, "We'll do things at your pace from now on." Nikki had been trying to lose weight, but that wasn't working very well for her. Still, she kept at it, hoping that one day it would pay off and she could have a kidney transplant and get off dialysis once and for all. She had been trying to lose weight for the last seven years with no success. We both agreed that I had to slow down from now on.

As we went back into the hospital, we stopped at the café for a coffee, then went back to the ward. I was getting a bit bored by this point. I'd been in hospital for three days now, with no TV to watch because I wasn't going to pay the high prices. One of the other men had already paid over £95 for his TV for five days. He had been in hospital for six weeks now and was struggling to keep up with the payments.

I wasn't going to pay that much for a TV that was on 24/7 while I was asleep. That was just stupid—a total waste of money. Not that I couldn't afford it, but it was the principle of it all. The whole thing was a rip-off, especially considering that the people who used it were vulnerable, ill people in the hospital for whatever reason.

Day 4

On the 4th day of being in hospital, the speech therapist came to see me. After a long chat, she told me that she was going to recommend I could go home, which put a big smile on my face. She gave me a lot of information on what I had to do when I got back home. She then said that I must slow right down and that Nikki would have to do more for herself. After that, she left me to it while she put her recommendations into the doctor at the hospital.

I looked over all the information she had given me, but it was very difficult to understand with my dyslexia. However, I knew Nikki would be able to help me with the bits I couldn't make sense of when she came to see me later. In the meantime, I saw the doctor who had been looking after me at the nurse's station just outside my ward. He had a long chat with the therapist and the nurses at the station, and then he came in to see me.

He asked, "How do you feel today?"

I replied, "Not too bad, I've been going for walks."

"Yes, I just heard," he said, pausing for a moment as he looked at my file. "The good news is you can go home tomorrow, but first we've got to sort out your meds."

"That's good news," I said. "I can't wait to tell my wife when she comes to see me later."

He added that I would still have to take it very easy.

"Yes," I said. "I fully intend to. Nikki will get used to it as I will have to."

He then left the ward, saying, "You were very lucky. It could have been much worse if you hadn't called 999 when you did. It could have been very bad indeed."

After he left, I went back to the information I had been given, trying to make sense of it all. But I couldn't. So, I left it until Nikki arrived that afternoon. Later that morning, I went for a walk again. This time, I had a bit of a spring in my step, knowing I wasn't going to be in hospital much longer. I had been bored senseless without a TV to watch, just listening to the other two men chatting about topics I had no interest in. All I could think of was going home that day.

Although I was feeling down in the dumps about my situation, the stroke, and the fact that I was so immobile compared to how active I was last week, before the stroke, I knew I had to be patient. I was moving so slowly now, and doing things was much harder. I had been told it would take time, but how long would it take? That was a big question.

That night, I went to bed, but I couldn't sleep at all because I was so focused on going home the next day. So, I sat up in bed meditating for a while. I find that it helps a lot until I was disturbed by a nurse who came to do my obs.

"What are you doing?" she asked.

I explained about meditating and how it helps when you need it. She did my obs and went off. I knew she would be back before the morning, and she was—twice! It's a good job I was only doing light meditation at the time.

Day 5

Just before dawn, on my last day in the hospital, I put my hearing aids in, and I could hear the birds singing outside the ward window. It was so nice to hear, until they were drowned out by the nurses clattering about just outside the ward. You could never get any decent peace and quiet in hospital; the nurses seemed to make noise all the time, and I'm sure they did it on purpose. Still, today I wasn't bothered, because I knew that I would be going home later, as soon as everything was sorted out and I was cleared to go. I couldn't wait.

The breakfast trolley arrived, and we all got stuck in. After breakfast, I sneaked outside for a smoke or two. It was a bit cold, so I was glad I had put trousers on under my dressing gown. The forecast for the rest of the day was sunshine all day, so that made me feel a lot better. After a while, I went back to the ward and got myself a coffee, as the others had already had theirs. I sat down in my chair by my bed for a while when Nikki came to see me. She had forgotten I was coming home that day, which was a bit unusual, given her memory loss since her operation, when I nearly lost her for the second time.

She stayed for about an hour or two. While she was there, the doctor came to check how I was doing and told me that I would be going home late that afternoon. When he left, I said to Nikki that there was no point in her hanging around, as I would make my own way back home.

"Are you sure?" she asked.

"Yes," I said.

"OK. Have you got enough money for a taxi?"

"Yes, I have more than enough."

She gave me a kiss before she went home, saying, "Love you, see you at home." I replied, "Love you too, as always."

I stayed on the ward until dinner time, then went outside for a bit. When I came back to the ward, I sat down with a coffee and started to pack up my things, examining my meds, which were locked up in the drawer by the bed. The next two hours dragged on and on. One of the nurses came to sign me out and gave me my meds from the drawer, telling me I could go as soon as she had got a porter to take me to the taxi.

"Thank you very much for everything you've done for me," I said.

"You're very welcome," the nurse replied as she turned and left the ward. It wasn't long before the porter arrived and took me to the front of the hospital. I thanked her as I got out of the wheelchair. She took the chair back, and I went outside to ring for a taxi. While I was waiting for it to arrive, I had a cigarette. It didn't take long before the taxi arrived, and the driver saw I was having a smoke.

"It's OK, you finish your cigarette first," he said. I gave him the thumbs-up. Once I stubbed it out and got into the taxi, he asked, "Where to?"

I tried to tell him my address, but my speech was letting me down badly.

"Do you want to write it down?" he asked.

"Yes," I said. I wrote my address down and explained that I had just had a stroke. Then, he understood, and off we went. Home and freedom felt like bliss. The thought of being back in my own surroundings was so good.

When I arrived home and got out of the taxi, the driver helped me to the door.

"I'll be OK from here, thanks," I said.

"Good luck," he replied, and drove off. I put my key in the door and went inside. I used the stair lift, and Nikki greeted me at the top of the stairs. She took my bag and said, "You go and sit down. I'll sort this out later."

I went into the front room and sat down in my armchair. As soon as I sat down, our two cats came over to me and were all over me. I guess they were pleased to see me. Nikki said they had been going nuts looking for me during the week I was in hospital. I said I could tell. When they finally settled down, Nikki gave me a coffee, and we sat down to have a long chat about the way things would be from now on.

I told Nikki that I had some information in my bag and that she should read it. I said there was a lot to take in, but we would look at it together later. In the meantime, I would write a letter to the DVLA to inform them that I had just had a stroke and was taking myself off the road until I received clearance from my GP to drive again. Nikki said we would do that later, but for now, I should relax. We had our drinks, and now I could have a cigarette whenever I wanted—no more sneaking out on my own for the long walk out of the hospital. I could just spark up whenever I wanted one.

I was on a long road to recovery. It was going to be weeks, if not months, before I could think about driving again. So for now, all I could do was look out the window at the car waiting for me to drive it, whenever that would be. But right now, I was in no condition to do much of anything, never mind drive safely. All I could focus on was my speech and my balance problems, which was going to be a very slow process.

Later that afternoon, Nikki asked, "What do you want to eat for dinner?"

I said, "Fancy a takeaway? What about Chinese?"

"Yes, I'd like that, but I'm a sloppy eater since the stroke," I added.

Later, we placed the order and set the table, which made it easier for me. When the Chinese food arrived, Nikki went to the door to collect it. When she brought it back, we took it into the kitchen to dish it up. Nikki said, "You go sit down, I'll bring it in." So, I went and sat at the table, putting my walking stick in the corner, and Nikki brought it in. We started eating, and it was nice—much better than the hospital food.

Although I was enjoying it, I was making a bit of a mess. Nikki said, "I see what you mean."

"Sorry," I said.

She reassured me, "It's okay. You'll get better as time goes on. Don't worry about it."

We finished the meal, and for the first time in a week, I was full. It was such a nice feeling.

Afterward, we sat down to let it all settle and watched TV. Nikki did the washing up, which was a first, while I flicked through the channels to find something decent to watch. I found a programme that had only just started. When Nikki finished the washing up, we sat down together to watch it. It was so nice to have no noise from the nurses in the hospital now that I was back home.

At about 9 pm, I was getting tired. Nikki said, "You can't be tired at this time of night."

I replied, "It's all part of having a stroke. Fatigue is part of it, but in time, that will get better."

"Okay," she said, "if you want to go to bed now, it's fine. I'll come in later, if that's okay with you."

I said, "Yes, see you in the morning," and went off to bed. Once I got comfy, it wasn't long before I was in the land of nod. Nikki came to bed later, and I didn't feel her getting in. We both slept in the next day, and it was about 7:30 when I woke up feeling a lot better for the rest.

1st Day Home

After I got up (which was late for me, but I needed it), I was very wobbly on my feet. But after a while, I managed to get into the front room. Nikki saw me get up and asked if I wanted a hand.

I said, "No, I'll be okay in a minute or so. Stubborn old git that I am, so independent." She just kept an eye on me to make sure I was okay.

When I got into the front room and went into the kitchen to make coffee, Nikki came in and said, "I'll finish that for you."

"Thanks," I said, as I turned to go back into the front room. I opened the curtains, looked down at the car, and thought to myself, *I wish I could just go for a drive.* But I knew I wasn't in any fit state to even think about driving just yet. So, I sat down, and Nikki brought my coffee in. The cats were meowing loudly, and I said to Nikki, "They're hungry."

"Well, we're very late getting up," she said.

"Okay," Nikki said, "I'll feed them." As soon as they had their food, there was total silence for a while.

I sparked up my first cigarette of the day, and we sat talking for a while about how I really felt about everything that had happened in the last week and how I was feeling now that I was home. I told Nikki how traumatic and horrifying it had all been and how lonely I had felt in the hospital. Even though she came to see me, I still felt like I was nothing. I couldn't speak enough to make myself understood. It took me so long to just go to the toilet on my own. It was very demoralising.

Now that I was back home, I still couldn't do much for myself. At this point, I could feel myself welling up. I couldn't hold it back any longer, and the tears started to roll down my face. Nikki came over to me and said how much she loved me and that we would get through this together. It didn't matter how long it took—we would do it together. After a while, I calmed down and drank my coffee. Just then, the cats came over and jumped up on my knee. After I stroked the cat for a while, I calmed right down. It's funny how a pet can make you feel at peace with yourself in seconds.

Nikki made me another coffee and brought it in. As she put it down, I said, "Sorry about that."

She said, "It was to be expected after all you've been through in the last week. Don't be silly. I told you I will always be here for you, just like you've always been there for me over the years."

Nikki then got the information from the hospital about strokes and how to deal with someone who's had one. She sat down and started to read it. After some time in silence, she said loudly, "Bloody hell!" which made me jump.

"Sorry," she said, "I didn't mean to make you jump, but there's a lot to know about strokes. I had no idea! Until you had one, I didn't realise. I see what you were trying to tell me the other day."

"We'll take things as slowly as you want to, and if you don't feel like doing something, we won't. Okay?"

I said, "That's okay by me. So from now on, we'll do things at my pace."

The annoying thing for me was that my life felt so damn slow, and I was having trouble coming to terms with it all. It felt like I was living in slow motion compared to how things were before the stroke. But I suppose I will come to terms with it in time.

Nikki said, "You have no choice. Just take one day at a time. Like driving—you will get there. It might take two months or so, but you'll get there."

She joked, "At least it won't cost a thing keeping it out there, will it?"

"No," I said with a bit of a smile on my face. "Yeah, I know. I'll still be able to look at the car in the meantime. At least while I'm waiting, the petrol won't cost me a thing. That's a change!"

"Yeah, but what I didn't think about was the extra money it was going to cost in taxis."

That afternoon, I took a short walk into the garden, and that was as far as I could manage for one day. To me, that was nothing— normally, I could walk for miles. But for now, it was one step at a time. I knew I would get stronger with time. So, we went back indoors, and I used the stairlift as stairs were a big problem for me right now. When we got back upstairs, I sat in my armchair and dosed off for a bit. Nikki let me sleep, even when I was snoring. When I woke up later, I felt so much better for it.

At about 5 pm, we had dinner and then watched TV. After that, we settled down for the evening until bedtime. I managed to stay up until about 10 pm, which was a more normal time for me to go to bed. When my head touched the pillow, I was out like a light.

2nd Day Home

When I got up the next morning, I still felt as rough as old boots, and I was still moving very slowly, as though I was dragging a heavy weight behind me. But I was told that it would get better as time went on, though no one could say exactly how long it would take. We would just have to wait and see.

Today, I made my own coffee and managed to get to the front room. Although I did spill a bit on the way, my coordination and strength in my left hand were still weak after the stroke, but they were getting stronger all the time. No sooner had I sat down to drink my coffee than the cats came over to see me. They were so good, and their charm helped keep me calm.

After breakfast, Nikki asked, "Do you feel like going out for a little walk today?" I replied, "I've got to get out and about. I'll give it a go later." Nikki said, "Okay, whenever you're ready," and we left it at that for now. I went on my computer for a while just to check on how my finances were doing. I managed to do that, but I was having problems with the keyboard. My hands just couldn't type properly, and I couldn't control the mouse very well either. I didn't stay on for long. I knew it would come back to me in time.

Later that day, after dinner, we went for a walk, and I managed to walk all the way around the block with my walking stick. We walked really slowly, but it made me feel so much better about myself. We stopped several times, and I was starting to feel a bit stronger. But one day at a time. As time went on, I was getting stronger bit by bit each day, so I just took it easy. I knew it would take a long time before I would be back to normal.

We went back home and had a coffee. As I sat in my armchair, we got talking about my recovery and just how long it was going to take. I said to Nikki, "I don't care how long it takes. It doesn't matter as long as I can get back to functioning normally."

"I just don't care," I added. "That time will come when it does."

Nikki said, "I'm not rushing you, but I am looking forward to when we can go back out in the car again."

"Yes," I said. "So am I, and it can't come soon enough."

"But for now, I'll just have to make do with starting the car now and again to keep it ticking over," I added. Then I said, "I want to have a shower at some point today."

Nikki said, "Okay, just let me know when, and I'll give you a hand."

"Yes, that will be nice," I replied, as I was still unsteady on my feet.

A bit later that day, I went for a shower, and Nikki gave me a hand. While I was in the shower, I stood up to wash my hair, and Nikki did my back. I stayed in the shower until my skin on my fingers went like prunes, but at least I felt so much cleaner. I got rid of that hospital smell and felt so much better for it. When I came out, I just put on my dressing gown for the rest of the day and chilled out.

I had a look at the info I'd received from the hospital, and it was an eye-opener, to say the least. That afternoon, I had a phone call from the speech therapist from the hospital. It was just a courtesy call to see how I was doing. While she was on the phone, I asked her what caused a stroke. She explained that the main reason was stress, and not just recent stress. She said that you might have had a lot of stress in your life, stress that you thought you'd gotten over, but your subconscious mind had stored it, and you'd forgotten about it all. You'd just got on with your life, but it was still there, sometimes stored in the back of your mind for years.

She told me that something in your brain starts it off, and it kind of explodes in your brain—that's how a stroke comes to cause you all the problems. And it takes a very long time to get over it. For some people, it takes longer than for others, but in my case, I had a mild stroke, so I should be over it in probably months rather than years.

Well, when I came off the phone, you could have knocked me down with a feather. I was gobsmacked at the thought that the stress in my life could have caused me to have a stroke. Nikki asked, "What's wrong?" She could tell by the look on my face. I said, "No, it's okay. That was the speech therapist from the hospital, and she's just told me the most common way people end up having a stroke."

I then went on and told her what the speech therapist had said to me over the last hour, but it took me over two hours to get it all out. Nikki then said, "Look at all the traumatic things you've been through in your life—broken marriages, losing all your children, and everything else you've been through."

I said, "Stop. I don't need reminding. Thank you."

"Sorry, I didn't mean to upset you," Nikki said.

I replied, "All that was in the past, and I don't want to be reminded of it, never mind talk about it."

"Okay," Nikki said, "I'll say no more for the rest of the day."

I just relaxed, and we said no more about my painful past. It took me a long time to push all those bad memories to the back of my mind, where I kept them over the years. But I knew I had to let them go for good.

So, I said to Nikki that I was going to go into the bedroom and meditate for a while. She said, "Okay, I'll leave you to it."

I got up out of my armchair, went into the bedroom, and closed the door and the curtains. The cats were asleep. I arranged the pillows how I wanted them, sat on the bed, got myself into the right position, and sat upright. I relaxed my mind, just like I had done so many times before, and went into a trance for the next two hours. I saw all the things that had gone on in my life and locked them back into the back of my mind, where they belonged. When I came out of the trance, I felt so much better.

When I came back into the front room, Nikki said, "Okay, now?"

I just put my finger over my mouth and said, "We won't say anything, okay?"

And that was that. We never spoke about it again. Case closed, as far as I was concerned.

3rd Day Home

I did not sleep very well the night before, so I got up at about 3 a.m. that day. I needed some early morning quiet time, and that's the only time of the day you can get it when there are no cars or buses and the birds in the trees were just starting to wake up. That time, just before dawn, I made a coffee and let the cats out of the night cage where they slept. They would come out when they were ready.

I sat down to drink my coffee and get my head back together. I loved that time of the day; it was so quiet, and it was a good time to hear the birds waking up. I would wait for the dawn chorus, which was so nice to hear in the mornings. It was also a very good time to work things out and solve problems you might have. By about 4:30 a.m., the birds were waking up, and you could hear them talking to each other in the trees outside. It was then that I would stand at the window, listening to them—pure bliss. Although I couldn't stand there too long now because of the stroke, it would be long enough for me.

At about 7 a.m., I could hear Nikki stirring, so I knew it wouldn't be long before she would be getting up. I went and made another coffee. I always had three before I went out in the mornings before my stroke, but now I was a man of leisure—for now, anyway. As I sat back down again, I nearly spilled all my coffee, but I stopped it just in time. At about 8 a.m., Nikki got up, all bleary-eyed, as she came into the front room and said, "Morning, what time did you get up?" I said, "About 3 a.m." "You're mad," she said as she sat down on the sofa and slowly woke up. We had a drink before breakfast.

After we had breakfast, I said to Nikki that I thought about going into town, as I was getting very bored being in all the time. She asked, "Are you sure?" I said, "Yes, if we take our time and take a taxi, I'm not up to going on the bus yet." Nikki didn't have dialysis that day, so we had all day to just potter around and take our time.

At about 10:30 a.m., we rang for a taxi and waited outside. It wasn't long before it arrived, and it was so nice for me to have a change of scenery. I could look around while we were going into town. I started off looking at the road for a change. When we got into town, I got out of the taxi. It was a bit low, but I just managed it. Then we went into the centre, and I had almost forgotten what it looked like for a while, but it all came back to me as we walked around the centre. It was coming up to lunchtime, and in the centre was the restaurant we liked, so we went in for a meal. As we went in, the staff we knew so well noticed that I was on a walking stick. I got a tray, and we told them what we wanted to eat. One of the staff asked, "What have you been up to?" I tried to tell them, but I couldn't get the words out, so Nikki chipped in and said, "He's had a stroke last month." The look of surprise on their faces was evident, and they said, "Sorry to hear that," as we went down towards the drinks section. Again, we were asked, and Nikki said that I had had a stroke. When we got to the till, the woman at the till said, "I'll bring it over for you," which was very nice. I had never had that sort of treatment before in my life.

We sat down to eat, with my face to the wall so nobody could see me eating. After we had finished, we sat at the table for a while. While we were sitting down, someone tapped me on my shoulder and said, "Long time no see." I looked up, and it was an old friend I knew from the Salvation Army. We had a long chat, and she said, "I'll let the people at the Army know what you are going through."

I used to be the caretaker at the Salvation Army in town. We said our goodbyes, and shortly after, she left, and we did too.

We went to some shops for a little while. I said to Nikki that I was getting tired and wanted to go back home. "OK," she said, as we made our way to the taxi rank just outside the centre. We had to wait for a bit, so I had a cigarette leaning against the wall. I just had time for one before the taxi came, and we went back home. I tried to have a chat with the driver, but he couldn't understand me until Nikki said that I had had a stroke not long ago, and then he understood me, as his dad had had a stroke two years ago and was still getting over it. He said, "I know what you're going through. I saw it with my dad." Just then, we had arrived back home. We got out of the taxi and went indoors.

I relaxed for the next three days. That little trip had wiped me out. Two days later, I went outside and got into the car just to start it up to keep the engine ticking over, as it had been sitting there for over two weeks. As I was sitting there with the engine running, my GP drove by on her way to work at the doctor's surgery just up the road. She waved as she went past. I thought, "I bet she'll ring me," and just a few minutes later, she did. She said, "I hope you're not thinking of driving." "No," I said, "just letting the engine run for a while. I know I can't drive yet, not for a long time." "Yes," she said, "another two months at least. Your speech sounds a bit better." "See you later," I said. "Bye for now." And then we went back home for the day.

4th Day Home

When I got up today, I was feeling okay. I made my coffee and sat down in the front room to give myself time to wake up, as I did the same every day. But today, I was feeling a bit better than I had in ages—much more confident than I had in some time, since before the stroke. I seemed to wake up quicker than usual. I just could not think of a reason for it, but I wasn't complaining. It was nice. It had been since the stroke first knocked me for six— that's a day I will never forget as long as I live, and I wouldn't wish that on anyone.

While I was having my first coffee, I wondered how long it was going to take and how long I would have to wait before I could drive once more. I was beginning to get frustrated with the time it was taking, but just then, I thought, "I just need to be a bit more patient. It will come in time." It was then I realised I was letting my mind get carried away, so I came back down to earth. I shook my head and said to myself, "Stop thinking like that. You'll drive yourself mad." So, I stopped thinking that way and decided to take the slow road to recovery. I had been thinking like that from time to time ever since I came out of hospital, and I knew it had to stop.

I got up and made my second coffee of the day and took it back into the front room. The dawn was just breaking, so I stood by the window and had a cigarette with the window open a bit. I could hear the birds singing in the trees opposite my home. It was so nice, and it always made me feel good about life again when I was down. It wasn't long before I was back to my normal self in my mind, at least.

I was getting a lot stronger now, and I knew that it wouldn't be that much longer before I could drive again.

About an hour later, Nikki got up, and I made her a cup of tea. I had my third coffee, and Nikki said, "How many is that?" I just said, "Well, I haven't had one since the last one. Ha-ha."

Nikki said, "You seem to be doing better than the other day."

"Yes," I said, "I feel a bit stronger today than yesterday and a bit more motivated. So, we'll go to town today."

Nikki looked at me and said, "What, like this?" She just had her nightie on at the time.

I said, "You can get dressed first if you don't want to be done for indecent exposure."

Nikki said, "You are funny," but she had a point as she pointed at my dressing gown.

I said, "No, I'll get dressed first."

Nikki said, "It's nice to see you're getting your sense of humour back."

Later that day, we went into town and took another taxi. We got dropped off at the park and went for a walk all the way around. While we were in the park, we saw a lot of people we knew, so walking all the way around took a lot longer than we thought it would. But I didn't mind; it was good to be in the fresh air all that time, to see all the wildlife, and the sun was out, which was very nice and warm too.

After about three hours, I was just feeling tired, so we called it a day and called for a taxi. We went back home, and I had thoroughly enjoyed the day. I thought I could find something else to do at home to keep my mind active. We had seen some adult colouring books in the shop the other day, and Nikki had dialysis the next day. So, Nikki said, "We'll see how I feel after dialysis."

"Okay," I said, "That's fine by me." I knew that sometimes Nikki didn't feel very well after dialysis, and sometimes, she was ready to go out straight away when she came back home.

5th Day Home

Today, when I got up, for once, I didn't have a fuzzy head like most days. Since the stroke, my head was nice and clear for a change, and I felt quite good about myself. While I was having my first coffee, I was totally relaxed. God, I felt so good today. It was wonderful. I was a bit later than usual, so as I sat down, I could hear the birds outside singing their little hearts out, and that just made me feel even better about life in general.

I finished my coffee and thought, "It's time I had another coffee, as I haven't had one since the last one." As I was out in the kitchen, Nikki came in and said, "Morning."

I said, "Morning," back. Then I said, "Do you want a cuppa?"

Nikki yawned and then said, "Yeah, please," still yawning.

So, I made her one and took it in, then I went back out to get mine. I returned to the front room with mine, sat down with Nikki, and we had our drinks while she woke up. We sat and chatted for a while before breakfast, deciding what we were going to do that day. Since it was a non-dialysis day and the weather wasn't too bad, I felt okay.

After we had breakfast, we got dressed and took another taxi into town. We had a look around the shops, then had a bite to eat, had a walk, and went back home. Just as we got home, I had a phone call from my GP. She said that my blood pressure was too high and that she had written a prescription for new blood pressure tablets—a higher dose to correct it—and she had sent them over to the chemist just up the road.

So, I put my shoes back on and went to get them. The chemist was just a short walk up the road, so it didn't take me too long. When I got back home, I said to Nikki, "Hi honey, I'm home," as if I had just come back from a hard day at work. "Can I take my shoes off again?" I sat down for the second time that afternoon.

I just relaxed for the rest of the day, as I was getting a bit tired after all the walking we had done the day before. I thought that I might be doing a bit too much too soon. I realised I was trying to run before I could walk, so I slowed down for the next week or so. I had been slowly going back into my old ways of doing most things around the house as a full-time carer, just like I had done before the stroke. That's because Nikki couldn't do that much for herself. I suppose that's partly my fault, where I had, without realising it, been taking over. Now that I was getting a bit better, Nikki just expected me to be able to carry on, but it wasn't long before Nikki realised that I could no longer carry on the way it was before my stroke. I was nowhere near as fit as I was back then. I had no choice but to slow down from now on, as hard as it was for me to do so. It will take time; I will just have to get used to it.

The trouble with me is that I have always been active all my life, and now I had to do the opposite. That is very hard, but I will just have to be more patient. I suppose in time, I will get used to it. This time before I can drive again is dragging on and on. It seems like I will never get there. I know I am getting very impatient. I have never had to stop driving for such a long time before.

1st Month Home

It has been five weeks since my stroke, and I am getting very fed up with doing nothing all the time. It's just not me. But now that we have the cats, they are giving me great comfort and making me feel at peace. It's strange how stroking an animal can feel so calming and relaxing.

As time went on, I felt much stronger, and each week that went by, I felt better than the week before. I started doing more for myself, but my speech was up and down. Some days I could speak quite clearly, and others it felt like my mouth was out of control, and I was speaking in slurred words. I was told to speak slowly so that my words would come out clearly and to help me regain control.

We were going into town a bit more often, and the taxi fares we had paid were mounting up. I was keeping a record of it, though I thought that might be a bit silly. You do daft things when you're that bored, anything to break the monotony of being laid up after a stroke.

Two weeks went by, and we hadn't done much. The weather had been so bad, and we had been stuck indoors except for Nikki's dialysis treatment three days a week. As for me, I was getting very bored and frustrated. The only time I was content was when Nikki was at home. I wish she didn't have to go through dialysis all her life, but there is some good news.

Nikki now has a living donor, and the donor is a perfect match. However, for the transplant to go ahead, Nikki has to lose another two stone in weight. She has been struggling with weight loss for years, so it might be a case of weight loss surgery, which Nikki isn't looking forward to. I can understand her reluctance, especially after already having two anaphylactic shocks and 22 surgeries in the past. She is scared of going through another operation after the last one, but she is now coming to terms with the idea.

We've both been to hell and back over the last 30 years of being together. Because we've been so strong for each other, we've pulled through it all. We've always faced things together and come out the other side better people. It's given us a much stronger marriage and a better understanding of each other. A lot of the people we know just can't understand how we've been together for so long and how we're still together after all we've been through. Where a lot of people would have drifted apart, not us. We're like a strong glue, unbreakable. I just tell people that love and respect for each other have a lot to do with it. No matter what life throws at you, you just sort it out. It's as simple as that.

2nd Month Home

It has now been three months since my stroke, and I feel like I am ready to start driving again. So, I asked my GP, and she called me in to see her. When I went to the surgery, she called me into her room for a long consultation, asking me a lot of questions. The outcome was that I would be able to drive soon, but I thought she was going to say, "Not just yet."

However, she said, "You are doing very well, considering you only had your stroke three months ago." She told me to take it easy, but I was fit enough. She asked me to wait in the waiting room for a little while, then called me back in. "I can see no reason why you can't drive," she said. "Just take it easy." I told her I'd just go around the block to start with to see how I'd feel. I thanked her, left the doctor's office, and went home to tell Nikki the good news. She said, "That's great! Maybe we can go out in the car later."

I said, "We'll see. I might try it on a short run while you're at dialysis, just around the block."

She agreed, saying, "Okay, but just be very careful."

When Nikki was at dialysis that day, I got into the car and took it around the block. It felt very weird at first, but by the time I had gone around the block, I felt confident enough to go to the garage and get some petrol. I came back home and waited for Nikki to return from dialysis.

When Nikki came in, she gave me a very surprised look and said, "Wow, you've been busy."

I jokingly said, "What do you mean? I've been sitting on my arse all morning."

Nikki laughed and said, "Yeah, right, it doesn't look like it."

By then, I was laughing too. I asked how she was feeling, and she said, "Fine. Want to go out?"

"Yeah, if you're up for it," I replied. "I feel better than I have in ages."

So, we went out, but this time we went to the harbour just for a change. We had a meal there, and it was a very nice change. We walked around the harbour for a while and watched the fish swimming in the water. We stood there for ages, mesmerized by them. Then we got back in the car, and I was feeling good about myself. I felt much more confident.

I was getting stronger now since my stroke, still using my walking stick from time to time, especially on long walks. I had learned to slow right down. I was no longer rushing about; I was taking my time, doing things at a much slower pace and living life with more patience.

3rd Month at Home & Driving Again

It has now been three months since my stroke, and I had been looking forward to driving again. I had been driving very carefully over the next week or two until my confidence returned to where it had been before my stroke. It felt so good to be back on the road again. Now I knew that things were getting back to normal.

Just before my stroke, my first book, *In the Mind of a Child*, was published, and I had just started my second book, *In My Mind*. So, my stroke couldn't have happened at a worse time. I had to put a hold on my second book until now. But with a bit of perseverance, I think I've made it. I've reached the goals I set for myself all those years ago. It has been a long time, but I've done what I set out to do.

The End

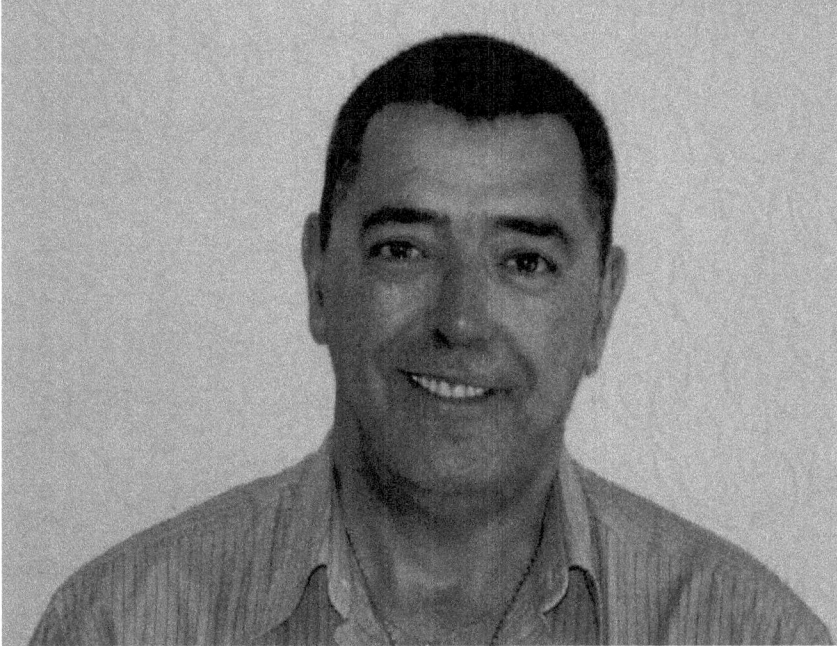

The Author of this Book

K. RAREHEART.

Live Well & Love Long

Be Happy with Life.

www.ingramcontent.com/pod-product-compliance
Lightning Source LLC
Chambersburg PA
CBHW071239020426
42333CB00015B/1545